MEN'S H

TURN FAT INTO MUSCLE

MEN'S HEALTH BEST

TURN FAT INTO MUSCLE

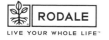

Every day our brands connect with and inspire millions of people to live a life of the mind, body, spirit — a whole life.

Edited by Joe Kita, *Men's Health* Magazine

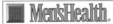
If you want to build muscle, improve your sex life, and do nearly everything better, visit our Web site at menshealth.com

Cover photograph by Robert Wright

Interior photographs
Beth Bischoff p. 36, 37, 42, 43 (top left, top right), 56, 57, 58, 59, 61, 63, 69, 72, 74, 75, 76, 77, 78, 79, 80, 81, 82, 83 ,84, 85, 86, 89, 90, 91, 92, 94 (bottom left, bottom right); Brand X Pictures p. 6, 9, 16, 35, 47; Corbis p. 38, 52; Image Source p. 55; Mitch Mandel p. 71 (top left, top right); Michael Mazzeo p. 41, 43 (bottom), 45, 45, 50, 51, 60, 62, 64, 65, 66, 67, 68, 70, 71 (bottom left, bottom right), 73, 87, 88, 93, 94 (top left, top right); Photodisc p. 18, 21, 22, 25.

Men's Health® is a registered trademark of Rodale Inc.

Printed and bound in the U.K. by CPI Bath using acid-free paper from sustainable resources.

Library of Congress Catalog-in-Publication data is on file with the publisher.
1–59486–260–5
Distributed to the book trade by Holtzbrinck Publishers
2 4 6 8 10 9 7 5 3 1 paperback

RODALE
LIVE YOUR WHOLE LIFE™

We inspire and enable people to improve their lives and the world around them
For more of our products visit rodalestore.com or call 800-848-4735

CONTENTS

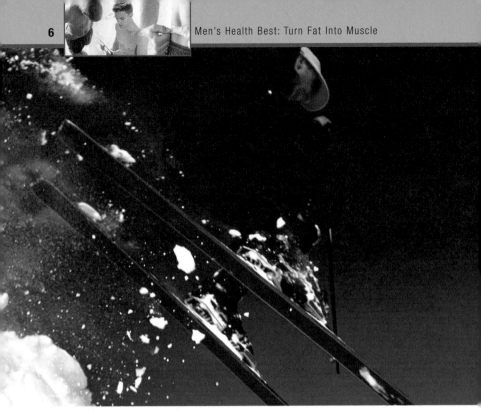

Living an active lifestyle is easier—and a lot more fun—when you're in shape.

INTRODUCTION

Let's be clear right from the start: You cannot magically transform fat into muscle. You're not going to go to bed tonight an average overweight man and wake up a preternaturally muscular male specimen. It just can't happen. But that's not what this book is about. What you will learn in these pages is how to burn that spare tire of a belly, those love handles that aren't adorable—no matter what your wife or girlfriend tells you—the wobbly double (or, God forbid, triple) chin that turns buttoning your top shirt button into an act of self-strangulation. And, as that fat melts away, we show you—with exercises and workouts that work—how to replace it with rock-hard muscles that were buried all along beneath all the jiggly stuff.

But first, congratulations are in order: Picking up this book is the first step on your journey toward unleashing the fit guy trapped beneath the body you see today when you look in the mirror. From this day forward, that fit guy is the image you must burn into your brain. Think of him whenever you

need a little extra motivation: He's the guy who looks great (even naked). The guy who *doesn't* wear a T-shirt at the beach. The guy who plays football instead of just watching it. The guy you'll be in (almost) no time, if you stick with the program.

We won't lie to you (that's what television commercials are for). It's not going to happen without a little effort on your part. But don't worry: We've made sure that it's nothing you can't handle.

How to Use this Book

If this is all starting to sound a little intimidating, don't let our enthusiasm worry you. The key to the changes you'll be making on the way to your goal is a commitment to consistency, not to extreme lifestyle changes. Here's how it works. In Part I you'll learn how to get started down the road from fat to fit with tips that actually recommend you not make too many changes at the same time. You'll learn how to deal with the various saboteurs in your life that get in the way of your losing fat and gaining muscle, like the television that keeps your butt glued to the couch and the friends who'd rather have a few beers after work than get some exercise. Then, of course, you'll get some nutritional advice, but it's probably not the advice you're expecting. We recommend that you eat more frequently rather than less frequently and practically demand that you include some good fat in your diet. Not only that, but we also advise that you always eat dessert. How's that for easy-to-follow guidance?

The Workouts

The heart of *Turn Fat Into Muscle* is Part II, the workout section. Take a look through it and then carefully consider which workouts are right for your current level of fitness— *not* where you'd like to be in 4 or 6 or 8 weeks or where you think you *should* be now. Read that sentence

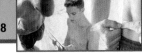

again. Most guys who start a new fitness regimen do way too much way too soon, get discouraged, and then give up. And where does that leave them? Disgruntled and, well, fat. If you've been down that road before (and most of you probably have), take a look at "Get Back in Shape," on page 46. It'll help you determine not only how to set your goals, but also where to start on your way to reaching those goals.

We know as well as you that the hardest part of any journey is the first step. It's probably the anxiety about starting that stalls most people. They hesitate, wondering whether they can actually pull off their grand goal. But we have the fix for that, too. *Turn Fat Into Muscle* includes several different kinds of workouts. This allows you to choose the one that works for you on any particular day, depending on what you want. Don't have much time to work out? Not a problem; we've included three quick and simple routines that you can do in 15 minutes flat. Ready to burn that fat? Turn to "The Ultimate Fat-Burning Workout" on page 38 for an 8-week program that will help you eliminate that oh-so-unattractive belly flab once and for all. And the best news of all? Every single one of the workouts included in this book does double-duty, helping you burn fat and build muscle at the same time.

Finally, *Turn Fat Into Muscle* ends with a section that illustrates and explains every single exercise that makes up the various workouts. We've left nothing to chance: Each exercise is accompanied by clear, four-color photographs, step-by-step instructions, and information about which muscles are being worked. In addition, expert Trainer's Tips explain how to make the exercises more or less challenging, depending on your level of fitness, as well as offering tips to make sure you're performing the exercises correctly to prevent injury.

And most important of all: Every last exercise, each piece of advice, every workout, has been developed by some of the world's top fitness trainers. Not bad for a 96-page book.

Turn Fat Into Muscle is a book that will never outlive its usefulness. You can turn to it again and again for advice about diet, health, nutrition, and exercise. And even after you've reached your goals, you can use the exercises and perform the workouts as part of your new, fit lifestyle.

So what are you waiting for? Put down the chips and step away from the beer. After all, there's no time like the present.

PART I:
Get in Shape

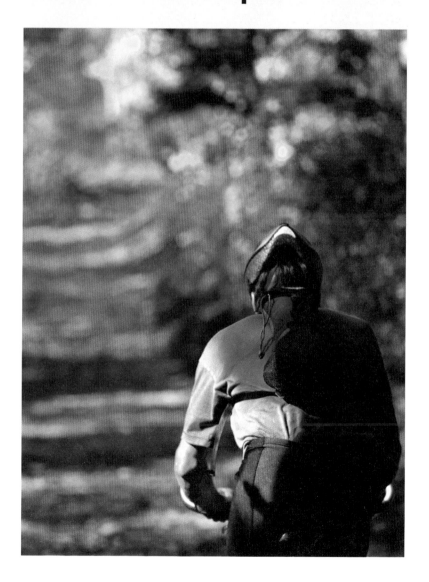

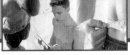

Getting Started

The hardest part of any journey is the beginning. The toughest step to take is the decision to get moving, to get started, to shrug off the comfort of inertia and get down to business. But the whole notion of getting in shape can be intimidating. Remember to keep things in perspective. Set clear goals, stay focused on the things you need to do to reach your goals. Here are some tips on getting started:

Stay encouraged. You don't have to exercise at a high intensity to increase your metabolism, build strength, or feel energized. Moderate activity yields these same rewards without the exhaustion. Exercise at a moderate intensity (breathing slightly harder than at rest) and you'll make steady progress. You'll reap a little endorphin high from even the lightest workout.

Work out when you can. You may have heard that morning workouts are better, since testosterone levels are higher. If you did, forget you ever heard it. The optimal time to work out is any time you can fit it into your schedule.

Do the workout, then cross it off. Mark an "X" on your calendar on the days you manage to get in a workout. Studies have found that exercisers who used this simple system of tracking workouts made more progress than those who didn't.

Stay with a program until it stops working. Switching too often from program to program can sidetrack your goals. Resist the urge to jump on every new workout routine you see; you'll make your workouts simpler (and see better results) if you stick to one program for 6 to 12 weeks, or until it quits working.

Figure out if it's working. If your waist tightens while your strength increases, you're on the right track. If you're not lifting more weight from one workout to the next, and your pants aren't feeling looser, the program isn't working. It's time to start making some changes.

Conquer one goal at a time. Don't try to get big, strong, and lean all at the same time—you'll end up splitting the focus of your workouts and falling short of any goal. Instead, pick one of the following goals, give yourself 6 to 12 weeks to achieve it, then move on to the next.

- **Get stronger:** Do one to five repetitions per set, increase weights by 10 percent a week, and again, cut back on cardiovascular exercise.
- **Get leaner:** Eat less, do more intense aerobic exercise, and try to maintain strength (it'll be hard to increase it) while doing sets of 8 to 15 repetitions with light weights.

Spend only 1 hour at the gym. The dropout rate is much higher when your routine lasts more than 60 minutes. Plus, you run the risk of breaking down your body more than you're building it up: Your body slows down its production of muscle-building hormones and cranks up the muscle-wasting hormones at about the 60-minute mark.

Simplify your schedule. Weight lifting any more than four days a week is too much, since the single best predictor of injury is how many consecutive days you work out. The more often you train, the higher your risk of injury—it's that simple. Try to divide your exercises into two balanced workouts—for example, upper body and lower body—and do each workout on alternating days. That way you train each muscle twice every 8 days, and give yourself plenty of time to recover from every workout, dramatically reducing your risk of injury.

Stay hydrated. Start the day with a liter bottle of water. Finish it off by the end of the day. Along with other beverages like milk and juice, that should keep you hydrated. Alcohol doesn't count—not only does it make you sprint to the urinal, it also dehydrates you.

TWO SIMPLE EATING RULES TO REMEMBER

Finding time to exercise can be tough, especially when you have to adjust your workout to your eating schedule. Here's an easy-to-remember guide to pre- and postexercise nutrition:

- Don't eat a big meal less than an hour before you work out. If you feel like you need something before you exercise, grab a carb-protein shake 5 minutes before your workout and sip it throughout the session.
- Eat carbohydrates and protein as soon as you can after your workout. The carbs help replace energy stores needed for your next workout; the protein repairs your muscle.

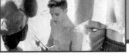
Meet Your Muscles

A good mechanic understands every inch of a car's engine before he starts tinkering with it. Before you start overhauling your physique, you should have a working knowledge of the major muscle groups that power your body. Each one of these muscle groups is addressed by one or more of the workouts that begin on page 35.

Chest

The *pectoralis major*—a large, fan-shaped muscle—covers the front of the upper chest. The chest is a primary muscle group that requires other, secondary muscle groups, mainly the shoulders and triceps, to assist in every exercise. If you work your shoulders and triceps beforehand, they'll quit on you before your chest works hard enough to grow. The smartest order is: chest first, shoulders second, triceps last.

Back

If you're looking for big muscles, there are none larger—when it comes to total surface area—than the ones in your upper back. The trapezius, a diamond-shaped muscle that runs from your middle back to your shoulders and then up to your neck, is targeted by the Snatch-Grip Shrug (page 69) and the Row (page 63). The lats run from your armpits to your middle back and provide the V-shape. Those large muscles are assisted by other muscles in your shoulders and arms, especially your biceps. The smartest exercise order: upper back first, shoulders second, biceps last—this way your shoulders and arms won't tire before you exhaust your upper-back muscles.

Arms

There's no point in getting scientific over arm muscles. The biceps bend your elbow, the triceps straighten it, and the exercises that target them pretty much repeat the movements. They do the job, but inevitably your arms grow accustomed to all that, and they stop growing. You need to confuse them. Switch up your arm workouts when they've stopped working (see page 10). Target different muscle groups and keep at it.

Abdominals

The abs include the *rectus abdominis*, the six-pack muscle, and the internal and external obliques, which are on the sides of your waist and assist in virtually every type of midsection movement—bending, twisting, crunching. (The *rectus abdominis* is mostly involved in crunching-type movements, but the obliques help out on everything.) Hidden beneath these muscles is the *transverse abdominis*, which wraps around your torso, attaching to your abdominals, pelvis, and ribs. It's a hard-working muscle that supports your entire torso, stabilizes your pelvis, holds your internal organs in place and prevents your gut from flopping over your belt.

Legs

Running, jumping, and heavy lifting all start with your hip, thigh, and lower leg muscles.

- The hip abductors, the outer-thigh muscles, move the leg away from the body.
- The hip adductors are the inner-thigh muscles. They pull the leg across the body.
- The hamstrings run up the back of the thigh and need to be loose for almost any athletic activity.
- The quadriceps make up the front of the thigh.
- The calves are located on the back of the lower legs.

ARE YOU FEELING IT?		
EXERCISE	FEEL IT IN YOUR...	BUT NOT IN YOUR...
Crunch (p.78–80)	Abdominals	Lower back, neck
Bench Press (p.70–71)	Chest, triceps	Shoulder joints
Biceps Curl (p.65)	Upper arms	Elbows, wrists
Lat Pulldown (p.76–77)	Upper back	Shoulder joints, arms
Lying Leg Curl (p.85)	Hamstrings	Lower back, gluteals
Row (p.58–63)	Upper back	Lower back, arms
Squat (p.88–90), Deadlift (p.66–67)	Thighs, gluteals	Knees, lower back

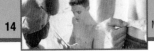

Your Fitness Strategy

You have a mission: Leave that extra flab in the past, and turn those soft muscles into steel. You've tried it before, but what went wrong? Assigning blame can be tricky. When your boss says, "We're not here to assign blame," duck. When we say you're not entirely to blame for your paunch, you're not off the hook, either. Nobody is the innocent victim of a drive-thru feeding. But there are sneaky factors—your friends, your family, your mindset—that can sabotage the best weight-loss plan. Your strategy: Identify the saboteurs, then adjust.

The Saboteur: Your wife

We do not suggest blaming her for your belly. This would be (a) wrong and (b) a reasonable defense at her trial. But researchers have found that men and women usually gain 6 to 8 pounds in the first 2 years of marriage. Once you're married, and that need to impress is gone, you may go to the gym less often, go out for meals or to parties more frequently, and develop new rituals, such as sitting on the couch with your wife and snacking.

The Fix: Reclaim that need to impress. Imagine what that girl at the gym thinks of your gut—or what she'd think if you had ripped abs. (Just don't hit on her.) And,

instead of diving into that bowl of buttered popcorn with your wife, ask yourself: Why am I eating? Is it boredom? Habit? Better yet, ask her to stop bringing those binge foods into the house. Establish healthful rituals. Instead of TV after dinner, take regular walks, or play a light game of basketball in the driveway. Any kind of light exercise suppresses appetite. Cool down with a sorbet (about 150 calories per cup) instead of ice cream (290 calories per cup).

The Saboteur: The baby

Dads-to-be gain almost 5 pounds from the end of their partner's pregnancy to the baby's first birthday. This phenomenon is especially common in young, stressed-out fathers. And the cycle repeats with each kid.

The Fix: Be a heroic provider, not a sympathetic eater. Prepare as if fatherhood were a sport—because it will be. Also, read her pregnancy books—they're full of excellent nutritional advice. As for her binge snacking and ice cream jags, adopt a simple policy, "She can have it, but I shouldn't." And, maintain your exercise routine—getting back into shape is going to be a lot tougher once your baby arrives.

FEED YOUR MUSCLES

If your buddy told you that drinking a glass of pickle juice would kick start your metabolism and help you improve your stamina in the bedroom, you'd probably accept the concoction and drink it down in earnest. Well, before you take that next swig, check out our roundup of some common muscle-building drinks and what they do—and don't do—to your body.

The Drink	Pros	Cons
Raw eggs	Eggs are one of nature's most intense forms of muscle-building protein.	Potential of contracting salmonella
Carrot juice	The human body converts beta-carotene into vitamin A, which strengthens the immune system. Carrots also contain B vitamins, vitamin C, calcium, and potassium.	When you consume too much carrot juice (about 3 cups a day), your skin can literally turn orange.
Pickle juice	It contains a lot of sodium; when you sweat, sodium keeps the body from dehydrating and cramping up.	It overloads regular athletes with sodium—it has 350 times the amount found in some sports drinks.
Wheat grass	It supposedly sucks nutrients from the soil and produces a variety of minerals, vitamins, and amino acids.	Your body doesn't need chlorophyll. Plus, this stuff tastes like a mowed lawn.

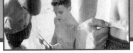

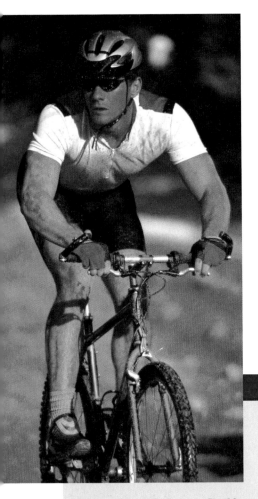

The Saboteur: Your kids

The presence of children in a household sharply increases the likelihood of there being junk food in the cupboard, and some of it is bound to end up in adult mouths. The same goes for stray fast-foods left over by finicky kids.

The Fix: If you discover yourself lurking around the house looking for remnants of your children's fast-food exploits, consider this: The sugary snack that a child will burn off during an hour of fidgeting will haunt you as a fat deposit. Read the nutrition label on any snack before unwrapping it. Realize the importance of setting a good food-and-

LOSE 10 POUNDS

Dropping a pound a week is safe, sensible, effective...and really slow. Luckily, there are ways to speed up the process.

To lose 10 pounds in...	Do this...
6 months	1-hour swim workouts two times a week
5 months	1-hour boxing workouts two times a week
4 months	1-hour cycling workouts three times a week
3 months	1-hour basketball games four times a week
2 months	1-hour runs five times a week
6 weeks	1 hour of stairclimbing five times a week
1 month	Have rough sex for 10 hours a day
1 week	Go for a walk—for 24 hours every day

exercise example for your children. Try to make junk food a once-a-week thing. Designate Friday as treat day. And instead of standing on the sidelines to watch your son's sporting event, volunteer to coach, ump, or ref. Make fitness a family thing.

The Saboteur: Your television

Not getting enough deep, non-REM sleep inhibits the production of growth hormone. This can lead to premature middle-age symptoms like abdominal obesity, reduced muscle mass and strength, and diminished exercise capacity.

The Fix: Try to mentally disengage yourself before you go to bed. Also, try doing your workout in the morning or afternoon—evening workouts may leave you too stimulated to sleep. Establish a ritual that signals your body that the day is over 30 minutes before bedtime—turn off the computer, read, stretch, or set the TV volume low.

The Saboteur: Your stress

Stress will spike levels of the hormone cortisol, which tells your body to store fat. And some people unfortunately appease their anxiety by reaching for fatty foods. Eating boosts insulin levels; combining that with cortisol leads to greater fat deposits. More stress, bigger belly.

The Fix: First, identify the type of stress you're under. Is it temporary, like studying for a bar exam, or more permanent, like your job? Short-term stress will pass. Long-term stress may require a permanent solution, like a new job. Make healthy eating effortless by snacking on foods that won't send insulin levels soaring: high-fiber energy bars or single-serving bags of almonds or cashews. Also, 15 minutes of explosive activity—hitting a speed bag or jumping rope—can alleviate anxieties and tension after work.

The Saboteur: Your friends

Buddies can make or break a diet or workout plan, whether it's unconscious scarfing of nachos during the game or the lure of pumping beers instead of iron. Worse, some of your friends might even deliberately try to sabotage your diet just for sport, with offers like, "Want a cookie?"

The Fix: Admit you need support. If you let people know how to help you, more often than not, they will. Eat a protein bar before meeting friends, so you'll feel fuller. When you're at the bar, drink a glass of water for every glass of beer. A time-tested strategy: Recruit a friend to diet or work out with you. Having someone to answer to is the best enforcement plan.

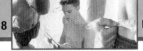

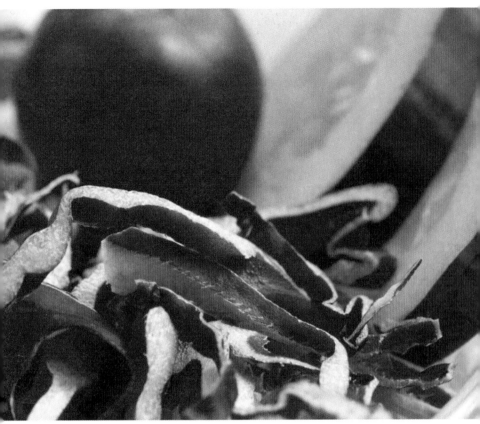

A diet that includes lots of colorful fruits and vegetables is a healthy diet.

Diet and Nutrition

Healthy eating is not as complicated as some nutritional experts make it out to be. Forget the jargon, the talk of carbohydrate-to-protein ratios, phytochemicals, and antioxidants—we have an easy way for you improve your eating habits. Here are a few simple tactics that will help you get more of the stuff you need into your diet while eliminating the stuff you don't. The best part? Before long you'll be dining like a nutrition expert, without even thinking about it.

THE BASICS

If you want to see your muscles, you have to get rid of what's hiding them. To do this, you must accomplish two simple dietary goals: Eat enough to preserve muscle, but not so much that you put on fat. Here are some basic rules to follow to lose fat and build muscle:

- Fill up on protein and multicolored vegetables. A high-protein diet makes you feel full longer and keeps your belly flat, whereas eating too many carbohydrates makes you feel bloated. Eat chicken, fish, or beef with as many vegetables as you want, the more colorful the better.
- Go easy on "dry" carbohydrates. After 4 pm, try to stay away from refined carbohydrates, such as white rice and bread. If you want to include a carb with your evening meal, choose the unrefined kinds, like wholewheat pasta or brown rice.
- Eat fiber. Fiber keeps you regular and helps your body better assimilate dietary fat. Try sprinkling your cereal with raw oat bran. Start with one table- spoon a day for two weeks, then double that amount.
- Consume good fats. Take in approximately 60 to 100 grams of fat per day, from avocados, olive oil, unsalted nuts, and peanut butter. A huge mistake some people make: They go fat-free and feel deprived. You must give your body good fats to feel full and satisfied.

Take your vitamins every morning. Evidence is mounting that a standard multivitamin fills enough of the gaps in your diet to make a real difference. A recent study showed that people who took a multivitamin supplement and 200 I.U. of vita- min E for 10 years were half as like- ly to get colon cancer.

Pile onions on everything. Research has revealed that onions are so healthful—they're a top source of heart savers called flavonoids— that it's practically your duty to eat them lavishly on hot dogs, pizza, burgers, sandwiches, and, of course, big green salads.

Drink iced tea. The more we learn about tea, the more healthful it looks. A single serving of black tea has more antioxidants—crucial to your body's defense against heart disease, cancer, and even wrinkles— than a serving of broccoli or carrots.

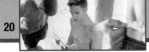

Eat a snack every day at 3 PM. A nutritional boost between lunch and dinner wards off fatigue and keeps you from overindulging later. Just don't scarf down a candy bar. Try yogurt and fruit, crackers and cheese, or eat an egg (hard-boiled), an apple, and a thirst-quencher like bottled water. All of these foods will give you long-lasting energy.

Leave the skin on your fruit. If you peel apples or pears, you're throwing away heavy-duty nutrients and fiber. Same goes for potatoes. Go ahead and peel oranges, but leave as much of the fibrous white skin under the rind as you care to eat—it's loaded with flavonoids. Ditto for the white stem that runs up the middle.

Eat red grapefruit. Remember lycopene, that stuff in tomatoes, watermelon, and guava that may fight prostate cancer? It makes tomatoes red, and it's responsible for the color in ruby red grapefruit.

Eat salmon once a week. Salmon is a rich source of omega-3 fatty acids, a type of fat most experts say we don't get enough of. Omega-3s seem to keep the heart from going into failure from arrhythmia—men who eat fish once a week have fewer heart attacks—and they may even ward off depression. A weekly serving of salmon should supply the amount of omega-3 fats you need.

Always wash your meat. Here's an easy way to cut the fat content of your secret chili recipe: As soon as you finish browning the ground beef, pour it into a dish covered with a double thickness of paper towels. Then put another paper towel on top and blot the grease. If you want to remove even more fat, dump the beef into a colander and rinse it with hot (but not boiling) water. The water will wash away fat and cholesterol. Using these methods together can cut 50 percent of the meat's fat content.

Eat broccoli with a little margarine, olive oil, or cheese sauce on it. This is our kind of nutrition advice. Broccoli is a rich source of beta-carotene—one of the major antioxidants your body needs. But beta-carotene is fat-soluble, which means it has to hitch a ride on fat molecules to make the trip through your intestinal wall.

EAT MORE OFTEN

Researchers in France studied the diets, weights, and body-mass indexes of a group of 330 men and found that those who ate small, frequent meals were significantly thinner and healthier than men who ate larger meals just once or twice a day.

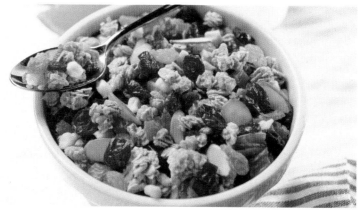

Breakfast *is* the most important meal of the day—and a bowl of whole-grain cereal is a perfect choice.

Without a little fat in the mix, your body won't absorb nearly as much beta-carotene.

Do a fat analysis before every meal. It's tempting to go fat-free at breakfast and lunch so you can indulge in a high-fat dinner. Not a good idea. Studies show that, for several hours after you eat a meal with 50 to 80 grams of fat, your blood vessels are less elastic and your blood-clotting factors rise dramatically. Research suggests that the immediate cause of most heart attacks is the last fatty meal, so, spread your fat intake over the whole day.

Always eat (a little) dessert. Sweets such as cookies and low-fat ice-cream bars signal your brain that the meal is over. Without them, you might not feel satiated—which might leave you prowling in the kitchen all night for something to satisfy your sugar cravings.

Eat a peanut butter and jelly sandwich just before you go to bed. A low-fat, low-calorie carbohydrate snack eaten 30 minutes before bed will help make you sleepy.

Diet Right

Diets generally fail for one of two reasons: Either they're too restrictive about the kind of food you put in your belly, or they too frequently leave you feeling as if you haven't put any food in your belly. In either case, it's usually not long before you have chocolate donut crumbs on the corners of the your mouth.

You won't be sabotaged by either of those problems with our program, which was created for us by expert trainers and nutritionists.

If you want to shrink your gut, get enough protein in your diet. In this case, about 25 percent of calories. Why? For starters, protein makes

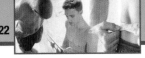

you feel full and helps you build muscle (which increases metabolism, thereby making it easier to lose weight) Just as important, high-protein diets have been shown to be the best way to attack belly fat.

Get enough fat. About 30 percent of your calories should come from fat. First, fat helps you feel fuller longer between meals, slowing your appetite. Second, it provides essential fatty acids needed for optimal health. Above all, fat makes you feel that you're eating real food, not starving in the land of plenty.

If you get enough protein and fat, your total calorie intake should take care of itself. Because you feel full, you won't binge on a bag of potato chips and blow your calorie count for the day. The remaining 45 percent of calories in our plan comes from carbohydrates—enough to give your palate a full range of tastes and your body a combination of fast and slow burning fuel.

These are all great reasons to pursue a healthy diet. But the best reason is this: Our program is an easy, sacrifice-free plan that will let you eat the foods you want and keep you looking and feeling better day after day. It's designed to help you lose weight by recalibrating your body's internal fat-burning furnace, by focusing on the foods that trigger your body to start shedding flab, and by rebuilding your body into a lean, mean, fat-burning machine.

Eating calcium-rich foods like dairy products and vegetables like broccoli can help burn fat more efficiently.

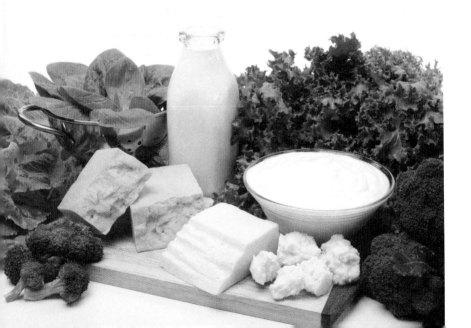

The Fat to Muscle Diet

The meals shown here are "templates" that you can vary any number of ways to keep your tastebuds happy. Follow them and you'll consume between 2,400 and 2,800 calories every day. That should provide plenty of calories for all but the most severely obese, while allowing most guys to shed fat from around their middles at a steady pace. (Don't worry about hitting all the numbers on the nose every time. If you exceed your fat quota during lunch, for instance, just cut back a little during dinner.)

Breakfast

- 1¼ c whole grain cereal or oatmeal
- 2 c fat-free milk
- 4 T almonds or other nuts
- 2 T raisins
  TOTAL: 591 calories, 29 g protein, 78 g carbohydrates, 18 g fat

Lunch

- Sandwich made with 2 slices whole grain bread, 5 oz lunchmeat or canned tuna, 1 slice low-fat cheese, 2 slices tomato, 1 T mayonnaise
- 1 carrot
- 1 c orange juice
  TOTAL: 666 calories, 41 g protein, 71 g carbohydrates, 25 g fat

Dinner

- 5 oz meat (pork, chicken, or turkey breast, lean beef, seafood)
- 1 c salad
- 2 T dressing
- 1 c dark green vegetables
- 1 slice or 1 c starch (bread, potato, pasta, rice)
- ¾ c fruit
  TOTAL: 379–952 calories, 23–53 g protein, 33–109 g carbohydrates, 12–43 g fat

Floater Meal

- 2 slices whole grain bread
- 2 T peanut butter
- 2 c fat-free milk
- 1 medium apple
  TOTAL: 629 calories, 31 g protein, 83 g carbohydrates, 20 g fat

RECIPE KEY

c = cup
T = tablespoon
t = teaspoon

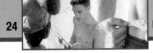

Essential Guide to Vitamins

Do something good for yourself that takes just 3 seconds: Swallow a vitamin before you go to work. On days when your diet has been less than perfect—no fruit and too much grease—the right combination of vitamins gets your body the essentials it needs. But choosing the right vitamin can be a pain in the neck. Have you gone to the store and tried it? You practically need a degree in nutrition to know the right combination of beta-carotene and thiamin and vitamin C. Most vitamins today are custom-formulated for specific conditions, and to get the maximum health benefits you have to pick the one that's the right mix for your needs—this can be quite tricky. We'll make it easy for you. No matter what your lifestyle, here's a guide to the right vitamins to take for your most basic needs—and most common complaints.

Heart Disease

If you have a family history of heart disease you need to load up on vitamins B6 and B12.

Research suggests that men with diets low in B vitamins are more than twice as likely to develop heart disease as men with higher levels of the vitamins in their systems. These B vitamins lower blood levels of homocysteine, a rogue amino acid that irritates the linings of your blood vessels, making them more prone to clotting.

Sun Exposure

To protect yourself from brutal sun rays all year round, make sure you get enough vitamins A and C, and lutein in your diet. Ultraviolet rays in sunlight break down vitamin A in your skin. Without that protective shield, you risk shriveling up and drying out by the age 40. A steady diet of vitamin A can help you build a reserve of the skin-cancer-fighting nutrients. You'll also need a solid dose of vitamin C; your body uses C to produce collagen, a connective tissue that keeps your skin and facial muscles taut. The lutein? It's for your eyes—helping to repair damage from the sun, so you won't have to squint while checking out the talent on the beach when you're 70.

Fight the Flab

If you're carrying around a few extra pounds, make sure you're getting enough of vitamins C, D, and E in your diet. Don't be fooled, lugging around all that extra weight isn't like doing the military press; it makes your bones weaker, not stronger. Getting your vitamin D, a crucial bone-strengthening vitamin, from a multivitamin can help. Finnish researchers found that men who took vitamin D reduced their bone-fracture risk by 25 percent.

Being overweight also increases your risk of diabetes. That's where vitamins C and E come in. Both protect blood vessels when your blood-sugar levels are out of whack.

Hangover

After a wild night on the town, load up on vitamins C and B1. Here's why: cigarette smoke—whether it's your own or someone else's—quickly burns up vitamin C reserves in your body, increasing your risk of lung cancer. Alcohol purges folate, vitamin B6, and zinc from your body. And we all know what a diet of vodka and wasabi peas can do to your liver. So down some vitamins C and B1 before a night of drinking; they'll help neutralize alcohol by-products in your system, significantly reducing the potential for liver damage when you imbibe heavily.

Stress Relief

If there's just too much on your plate, try taking a vitamin that includes choline, magnesium, and vitamin K. Recent research suggests that choline—a well-known stress fighter—improves memory and helps cells in the brain communicate better. A good multivitamin can also make up for the magnesium and vitamin K deficiencies you can get from living on take-out food and frozen microwave meals.

Build More Muscle

If you're trying to bulk up, take chromium and vitamins B6 and B12. Why? Chromium improves your

The right multivitamin can relieve and prevent a whole host of complaints.

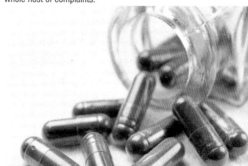

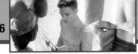

body's ability to convert amino acids into muscle. Research suggests that men who exercise regularly and take 200 micrograms of chromium a day add more muscle weight and lose significantly more body fat than

Essential Vitamins

VITAMIN	FAT SOLUBLE	WATER SOLUBLE	SOURCE
A	X		Pumpkin, carrots, sweet potatoes, beef liver, most dark green leafy vegetables, eggs and cheese
B6		X	Nuts, legumes, eggs, meats, fish, whole grains, and fortified breads and cereals
B12		X	Seafood, poultry, meat, and dairy products
C		X	Citrus fruits, red and green peppers, brocc orange-fleshed melon, and strawberries
E	X		Wheat germ, corn, nuts, seeds, olives, gree leafy vegetables, and vegetable oils (such corn, sunflower, soybean, and olive oil)
Folate		X	Whole grains, most dark green leafy vegetables, citrus fruits, poultry, and fortifi breads and cereals
Niacin		X	Enriched whole-grain cereals, chicken, fis beef liver, veal and pulses
Pantothenic acid		X	Eggs, fish, dairy products, whole-grain cereals, legumes, yeast, broccoli, and othe vegetables in the cabbage family
Riboflavin		X	Lean meats, eggs, legumes, nuts, green le vegetables, dairy products, milk, and fortif breads and cereals

lifters who don't take these supplements—hard workouts deplete your B vitamins. Below is more information about some essential vitamins and their effects on the body.

FUNCTION
Helps in the formation and maintenance of healthy teeth and skeletal and soft tissue; essential for healthy eyes and skin; regulates the immune system.
Needed for normal brain function, energy production, and to metabolize protein. The higher the protein intake, the greater the need for vitamin B6.
Plays an important role in the formation of red blood cells, maintenance of the central nervous system, and metabolism.
An antioxidant that protects your body from free radicals, which may cause heart disease and cancer. Also helps your body to absorb iron effectively.
Important in the formation of red blood cells; acts as an antioxidant to protect body tissue from the damage of oxidation.
Helps in the production and maintenance of red blood cells. It also helps prevent anemia, osteoporosis-related bone fractures, and changes to DNA that may lead to cancer.
Helps in the functioning of the digestive system, skin, and nerves. It is also important in energy metabolism.
Also known as vitamin B5. Is essential for the metabolism of food, as well as for the synthesis of hormones and cholesterol.
Important for body growth and red blood cell production, and helps release energy from carbohydrates.

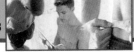

The Benefits of Stretching

Some men are so crunched for time that they just want to get their workout over with as quickly as possible. Doing a quick warm-up to loosen your muscles and get the blood flowing, followed by a few minutes of stretching can be enormously beneficial to your workout. Just five to seven minutes of stretching before and after exercise will increase flexibility. Stretching prevents injury and soreness, helps free your body of muscular tension, improves circulation, and enhances muscle tone—giving your muscles a more defined look.

CROSS STRETCH

Stand with your feet shoulder-width apart and your knees slightly bent. Lift your arms so they form a "T" with your torso, and turn your palms down. Slowly rotate your thumbs backward and stick out your chest as you pull your arms back. Pinch your shoulder blades together to extend your range of motion. Now, instead of holding one long stretch, do five pulsing stretches. That is, pull your arms back an extra inch or two, and then allow them to spring forward an inch or two; repeat.

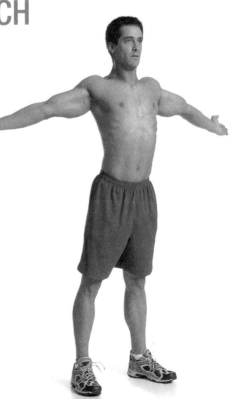

UPPER-BACK STRETCH

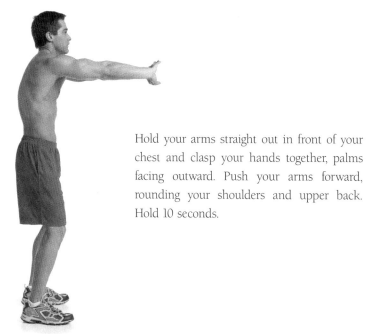

Hold your arms straight out in front of your chest and clasp your hands together, palms facing outward. Push your arms forward, rounding your shoulders and upper back. Hold 10 seconds.

SHOULDER AND NECK STRETCH

Place both arms behind your back and grab your right wrist with your left hand. Tilt your head to the left and pull your right arm to the left. Hold for 10 seconds, and then repeat on the other side.

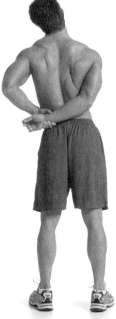

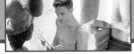

LOWER-BACK STRETCH

This stretch resembles a reclining spread eagle. Lay flat on your stomach. Slowly lift your upper chest, shoulders, neck, and head. Be sure not to strain your neck. As you are doing this, also stretch and lift your lower legs and feet a few inches above the ground. Keep your hands behind you and extend them, with fingertips straight out. Stretch your body from head to toe. Hold for 15 seconds per repetition. Work up to one or two sets of eight repetitions.

HOW OFTEN SHOULD I STRETCH?

If you're stuck behind a desk all day, stretch every few hours to avoid back and shoulder tightness that comes from hunching over a keyboard. Perform the Chest Stretch on page 32 to open your chest and relax your shoulders and back. To stretch your glued-to-the-chair glutes, cross your left leg over your right, resting your left ankle on your right knee. Bend forward at the waist and hold the stretch for 10 seconds. Then switch legs and repeat.

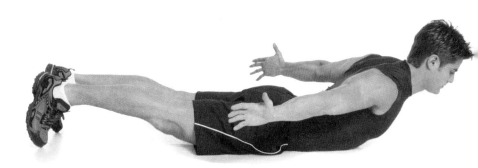

GROIN STRETCH

Sit on the floor and place the soles of your feet together. Grasp your ankles and gently push your knees down with your elbows. Hold for 10 seconds. You will feel this stretch in your inner thighs.

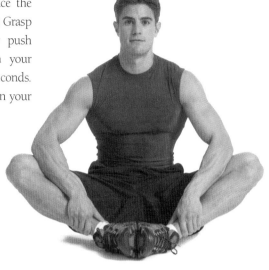

SPINAL-ROTATION STRETCH

Lie flat on your back with your arms out to your sides, forming a "T" with your body, and turn your palms toward the ceiling. Your feet should be flat on the floor, your knees bent and resting against each other. Now slowly roll your lower body to the right as one unit, keeping your knees, lower legs, and thighs together and your arms flat on the floor. Turn your head to the left. Breathe normally while you hold the stretch for 15 to 30 seconds. You should feel a gentle release in the muscles of your lower back. Repeat, turning your lower body to the left and your head to the right. Complete three repetitions on each side. If this hurts, stop immediately.

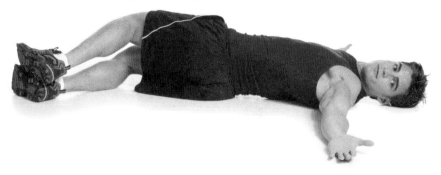

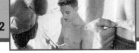

CHEST STRETCH

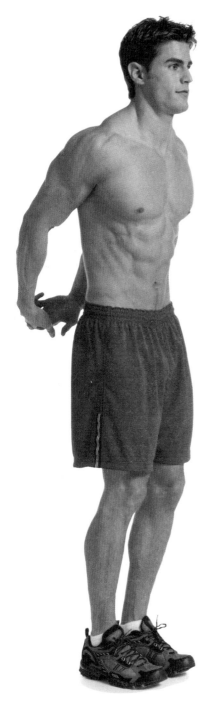

Clasp your hands together, palms up, behind your lower back. Pull your arms up toward your head. Hold for 10 seconds.

LYING ILIOTIBIAL BAND STRETCH

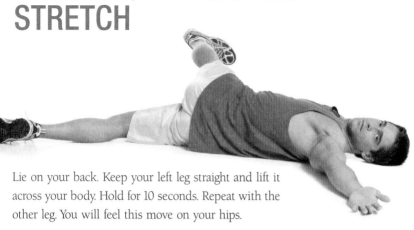

Lie on your back. Keep your left leg straight and lift it across your body. Hold for 10 seconds. Repeat with the other leg. You will feel this move on your hips.

MODIFIED-LUNGE STRETCH

Find a padded surface and kneel on your left knee with your right leg extended straight out in front of you, toes up, and heel on the floor. Keeping your left hand on the floor for balance, lean forward, shifting weight to your right foot, and grab the toes of that foot with your right hand. Pull the toes toward you and feel the stretch in the back of your right leg. You should also feel a mild stretch in the front of your left thigh. Hold for about 30 seconds (or longer), and then relax. Alternate legs and repeat. Do three to five with each leg.

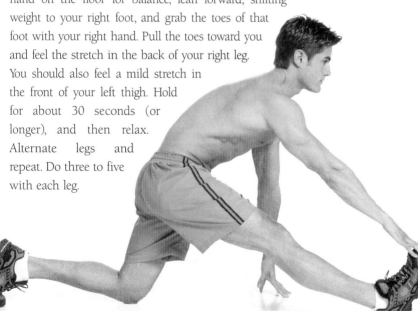

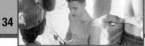

FULL-BODY STRETCH

End every workout with this move: Sit on the floor with your left leg straight out in front of you. Bend your right leg and put the sole of your right foot against the inside of your left thigh. (Your legs will look like the number 4.) With your left hand, try to touch either your left ankle or your left big toe. This stretches your left calf, Achilles tendon, hamstring, hip, knee, glutes, lower-back muscles, shoulder, and wrist. Hold the position for 30 to 60 seconds, then switch sides.

BE FLEXIBLE

Flexibility is the easiest fitness element to develop. As with other types of training, improvement in flexibility depends on subjecting muscles to more than they're accustomed to by working them through a range of motion in a controlled and systematic way. You merely need 10 extra minutes or so to what you already do.

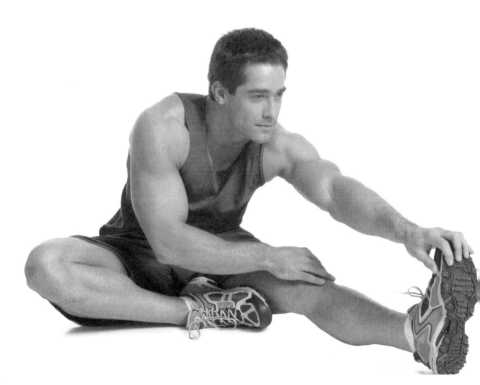

PART II:
Ultimate Workouts

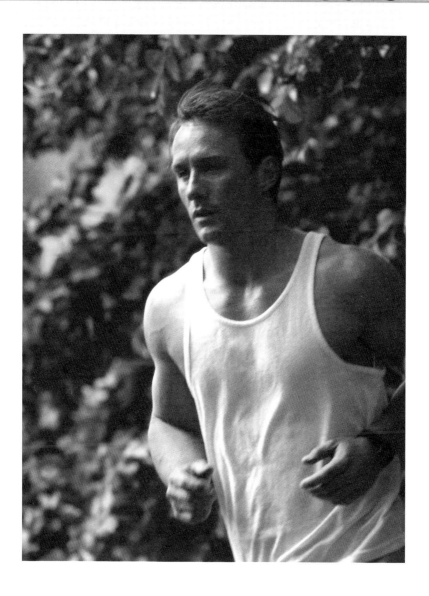

Fat to Fit Workout

Keep your muscles awake with this 4-week fat-burning program from Tim Kuebler, C.S.C.S. Do four sets of ten repetitions of each exercise. Rest 60 seconds between sets, 3 minutes between exercises, and a day between workouts. Do this routine 3 days a week.

UNEVEN STEP SQUAT

Targets: Entire Lower Body

DAY 1: Stand with a barbell resting on top of your shoulders, with your left foot on an exercise step and your right foot to the right of the step. Lower your body until your right thigh is parallel to the floor. Pause, then return to the starting position. Do one set this way, then switch sides.

DAY 2: Same as Day 1, but explode upward so that the foot off the step leaves the floor.

DAY 3: Same as Day 2, but alternate legs on each rep: move from one side of the step to the other.

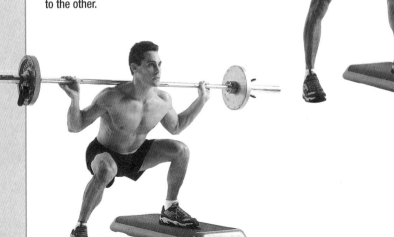

WALKING JERK LUNGE

Targets: Entire Lower Body, Deltoids, Trapezius

DAY 1: Stand holding an EZ-curl bar overhead. Step forward with your left leg so that its thigh is parallel to the floor and your knee is over (not past) your toes. As you bring your right leg up even with the left, lunge forward with your right leg. Alternate legs until you complete the set.

DAY 2: Same as Day 1, but hold the bar at your collarbone, pressing it up as you lunge forward. Lower it as you bring your feet together.

DAY 3: Hold a pair of dumbbells out to your sides, with palms facing you, as you lunge forward with your left leg; lower them as you bring your feet together.

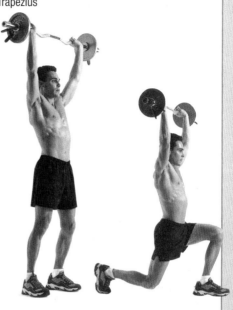

BASEBALL SWING

Targets: Obliques

DAY 1: Stand holding a 5-pound plate or dumbbell with both hands, your arms in front of you at chest level. Swivel your torso to the right as far as you can, then to your left as far as you can. Continue this movement for 10 seconds, then increase your speed for 20 seconds.

DAY 2: Same as Day 1, but move the weight in a sideways figure-eight motion.

DAY 3: Same as Day 2, but sit on the floor with your legs bent and feet flat on the floor, and lean back from the hips at a 45-degree angle.

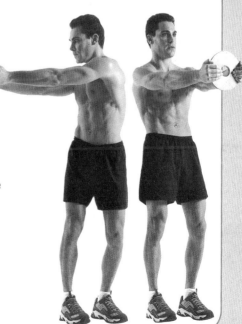

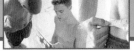

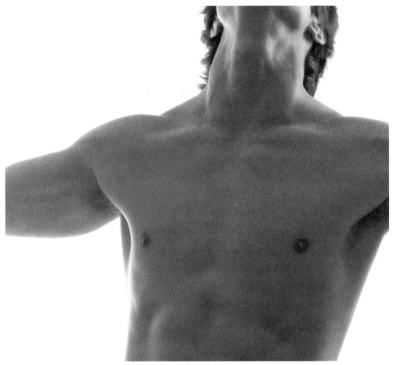

Burn away those excess pounds and taking off your shirt won't be such a nightmare.

The Ultimate Fat Burning Workout

Here's an 8-week workout program designed to help you attack the excess flab hanging around your middle once and for all. No fancy dieting gimmicks, electronic gizmos, or miracle pills—just a simple, instinctive, and satisfying eating and exercise plan that will produce serious, long-lasting results. As soon as you start expending more calories than you take in, you'll start burning stored fat for energy. With the diet changes and this exercise program, you could lose a pound or two of fat each week for 8 weeks.

Your Fat-Burning Workout

You'll train your body with three different routines each week (see charts on the next page). This ensures that your muscles will take longer to get used to each series of exercises and work harder to make adaptations. Training in this way elevates metabolism, helping you burn more calories between workouts.

- **Monday Routine:** Do 10 repetitions of each exercise in a circuit—that is, do one set of every exercise before repeating any of them. Start with a warmup circuit, using one-half to two-thirds of the weight you'll use in your actual work circuits. Then do one, two, or three circuits, depending on your experience, fitness level, and time allotted. If you're a total beginner, aim for one or two circuits the first week, and gradually build up to three circuits.
- **Wednesday Routine:** Do 15 repetitions of each exercise in a circuit. Start with a warmup circuit, using one-half to two-thirds of the weight you'll use in your work circuit. Then do one work circuit. Finish by doing the aerobic routine (see box page 41).
- **Friday Routine:** Do 10 repetitions of each exercise. Start with a warmup set, using one-half to two-thirds of the weight you'll use in

your work sets. Then do three consecutive sets of each exercise before moving on to the next exercise.

Stretching Essentials

Don't dive right into your weight-training workout—stretch before you train, and warm up before you stretch. Do about 10 minutes of low-intensity exercise on a stationary bike or a treadmill to decrease the chance of injury and to elevate your body temperature before your workout. Once your muscles are warm, stretch them for another 5 to 10 minutes, focusing on the body parts you plan to train. To help prevent muscle soreness after your workout, cool down with light aerobic exercise for about 5 minutes and then stretch for another 5 to 10 minutes.

Weight Lifting Basics

If you've never lifted before, trial and error can determine the amount of weight you'll lift in each exercise. Try to increase the amount by about 10 percent each week.

Your Diet Plan

A healthy, balanced diet combined with a targeted exercise program is still the best ticket to permanent total-body fat loss. For tips about how to diet safely, and for a sample meal plan see page 23 in Part I.

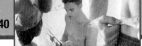

Monday Routine

EXERCISE	REPS
Barbell squat (p.89) 50 40	10
Barbell bench press (p.71) 40	10
Farmer's walk on toes (p.93) 20	10
45-degree traveling lunge (p.87) 20	10
Wide-grip seated row (p.62) 80	10
Swiss ball crunch (p.79)	10

Wednesday Routine

EXERCISE	REPS
Leg press (p.84)	15
Good morning (p.94)	15
Wide-grip barbell bench press (p.71) 20 25	15
Towel pulldown (p.77) 60 75	15
45-degree lying dumbbell row (p.61) 15 20	15
Towel crunch (p.80)	15

Friday Routine

EXERCISE	REPS
Dumbbell split squat (p.89)	10
Romanian deadlift (p.67)	10
Twisting shoulder press (p.56) 20	10
Pushup bridge (p.83)	10
One-arm lat pulldown (p.77)	10

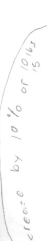

Decrease by 10% or 10 lbs

AEROBIC ROUTINE

Instead of performing long, slow, steady aerobic exercise, go hard for short periods, then easy for a minute or two. Do the cardiovascular workout one to three times a week.

- Do any type of aerobic exercise you like, one to three times a week after lifting.
- Warm up for 5 minutes by going at a very easy pace, gradually increasing your effort until you're at 50 percent of your maximum.
- Go as hard as you can for 15 seconds.
- Recover for 2 minutes, returning to the pace at which you finished your warmup
- Start the next interval and do a total of six to 10 intervals.
- After your last 2-minute recovery, go at an even easier pace for 3 minutes to cool down.

THE 15-MINUTE WORKOUT

Lift, Jump, Lift

Nothing burns fat as quickly, or efficiently, as an intense cardio-and-weights circuit. Adding a simple rope-jumping component to your routine makes a world of difference—10 minutes of jumping rope burns as many calories as 30 minutes of running. So dust off your old jump rope and give this a try—the pounds will melt away faster than you can count them.

DUMBBELL DEADLIFT

Targets: Gluteals, Hamstrings, Quadriceps

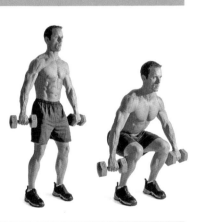

1. Stand with your feet shoulder-width apart and grasp a pair of dumbbells with an overhand grip, holding them down at arm's length at your sides.

2. Bend your knees and your hips—but don't bend your back—and lower your body until your thighs are parallel to the floor.

3. Stand, thrusting your hips forward and keeping your shoulders pulled back. Repeat.

ABOUT YOUR WORKOUT

Perform the deadlift with a weight you can lift eight times at most, and do six repetitions. Without resting, jump rope for 45 seconds. Then do the push-press, followed by 45 seconds of rope jumping. Do three more circuits and decrease the weight by 20 percent each time. Complete the four circuits in 15 minutes.

PUSH-PRESS

Targets: Deltoids, Triceps

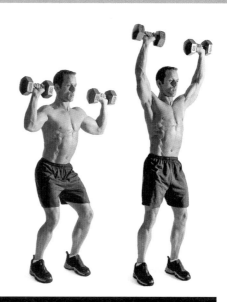

1. Stand with your feet shoulder-width apart and knees slightly bent. Hold the dumbbells at jaw level, as if ready to press them over your head.

2. Bend your knees slightly to dip your body, then push up with your legs as you press the dumbbells overhead. Keep your torso upright throughout.

3. Lower dumbbells to starting position. Repeat.

JUMP LIKE A PRO

Sure, you did it all the time as a kid, but jumping rope is not as simple as you think. Reaping the full rewards of this cardiovascular exercise requires some skill and practice. Here are a few pointers:

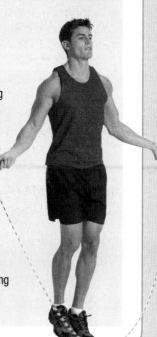

- Balance your weight on the balls of your feet, keeping your knees slightly bent. Don't jump higher than an inch. Keep your body upright, eyes front, and elbows close, and make small circles with your wrists.

- As you jump, push through the floor with the balls of your feet and point your toes downward. The jump should come from the ankles, calves, knees, and hips.

- Land softly by spreading the impact through your ankles, knees, and hips. Contact with the ground should be as brief as possible, your heels never touching the ground. Don't double bounce. That's too easy.

THE 15-MINUTE WORKOUT

Lose Your Layers

Shed that stubborn roll around your middle with this powerful fat-loss workout. Perform the workout below 3 days a week, incorporating the variations on days 2 and 3. The variations ensure that you work your muscles in a slightly different way each time, which forces you to work harder while strengthening your body at every angle—this is key in preventing sports injuries. Do the exercises as a circuit, moving from one to the next without rest. Complete a total of four circuits, resting 60 seconds after each.

GOLF SQUAT

Targets: Entire Lower Body, Deltoids

Day 1: Hold one 20-pound dumbbell with both hands at arm's length in front of your body, your upper arms pressed against your chest. Keep your torso upright and lower your hips until your thighs are at least parallel to the floor. Pause 1 second, then rise to a standing position as you rotate your upper body to the left and lift the weight toward the ceiling, keeping your arms straight as if swinging a golf club. Lower the weight as you return to the starting position. Repeat, this time rotating to your right. Do 15 repetitions on each side.

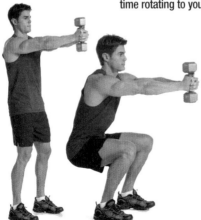

Day 2: Perform the same move with two light dumbbells, holding one in each hand. As you stand up and rotate to the left, keep your right arm down while lifting your left arm toward the ceiling. As you rotate to the right, keep your left arm down and lift your right arm toward the ceiling.

Day 3: Same as day 2, but as you lift one arm, punch across your body with the other.

BROAD JUMP

Targets: Entire Lower Body

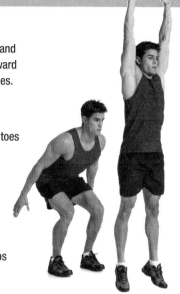

Day 1: Stand with your feet shoulder-width apart and knees slightly bent. Dip your knees and jump forward as far as you can. Land on both feet with soft knees. Pause, then jump again. Complete a set of 10.

Day 2: Hop forward about 2 feet. As soon as your toes touch the floor, jump again. Complete a set of 10.

Day 3: Same as day 1, but after each broad jump, squat slightly and quickly explode straight up, reaching both arms overhead (as shown). Land with soft knees, then jump forward again. Complete a set of 10 broad jumps with a vertical jump after each.

SWISS BALL PUSHUP

Targets: Pectorals, Triceps, Front Deltoids, Midsection Stabilizers

Day 1: Get into pushup position with your shins on a Swiss ball and your hands on the floor. Do 20 standard pushups.

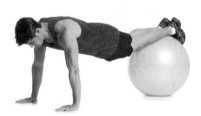

Day 2: Same as day 1, but lift one leg off the ball and do 10 pushups. Change legs and do another 10.

Day 3: Same as day 1, but move your hands out so they're 6 inches farther apart than normal.

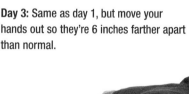

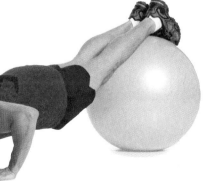

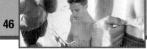
Get Back in Shape

Take out a tape measure. Measure your waist around the belly button. Now suck in your waist until it's 2 inches smaller. That's what the average guy gets on this program. If you've recently fallen off the fitness wagon, or even if you've never really been able to stick to a workout routine, here's your chance to get back on track and shed those excess layers.

Identify Your Goals

What's the first thing most of us do to get back into shape? We run out and join the gym, buy another piece of expensive workout equipment, or maybe even go so far as to hire a personal trainer. All before we've figured out what we want or expect from our new workout regimen. The first thing you need to do is figure out what your goals are—and the more specific the goal, the more likely you are to start working toward it and ultimately reach it. Instead of, "I want to get in shape and lose weight," make your goal: to lose 2 inches off your waist or drop 10 pounds. Once you have a specific goal, the next step is to give yourself time to accomplish it. Tell yourself you're going to lose 2 inches or 10 pounds in 6 to 8 weeks.

Make a Plan

Remember that all exercise is good for something, but not every exercise is good for everything. If you want to lose inches, combine weight training, cardiovascular exercise, and a smarter diet. A 1999 study found

	WEEK 1		
EXERCISE	WEIGHT	REPS	
Dumbbell squat (p.88)	15	15	
One-arm bent-over row (p.59)	20	15	
Pushup (p.72)	Body	15	
Shoulder press (p.56)	15	12	

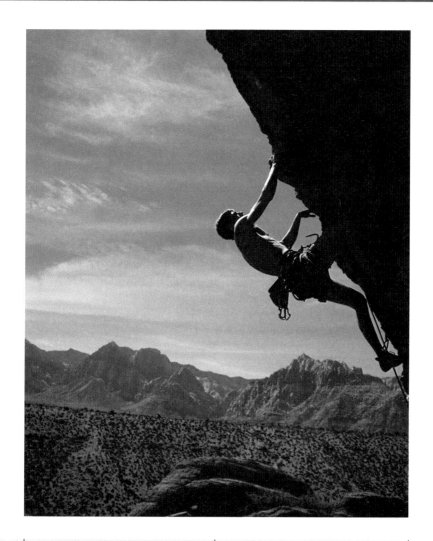

WEEK 2		WEEK 3	
WEIGHT	REPS	WEIGHT	REPS
20	12	20	12
25	12	25	12
Body	20	Body	20
20	12	20	12

	WEEK 4		
EXERCISE	WEIGHT	REPS	
Dumbbell stepup (p.91)	15	12	
One-arm bent-over row (p.59)	25	12	
Decline pushup (p.73) **	Body	12	
Shoulder press (p.56)	20	12	

** During Week 4 do a regular pushup (p.72)

	WEEK 7		
EXERCISE	WEIGHT	REPS	
Dumbbell lunge (p.86)	15	8	
One-arm bent-over row (p.59)	40	8	
Dumbbell bench press (p.70)	30	10	
Shoulder press (p.56)	25	10	

that guys who did all three lost 22 pounds in 12 weeks, and virtually all the weight lost was fat. If you want to lose pounds, focus on food and aerobic exercise. Although, when it comes to losing weight, diet gets you there faster. Here's why: Walking or running a mile burns roughly 100 calories. To lose a single pound of fat, you need to burn 3,500 calories. That's 35 miles per pound, or almost a marathon and a 10-miler combined. That'll make the turkey sandwich go down easier, right?

If you want to build strength, hit the weight room. Also, avoid severe calorie deficits and too much cardiovascular exercise. Both of these can lower your testosterone levels, making it more difficult to build strength.

If you want to prepare for a sport, work on devloping specific skills and the type of endurance the sport requires. For example, basketball requires short bursts of speed; running long distances slowly won't prepare you for that.

Start at the Halfway Point

During the first week of your new workout program, train only half as hard as you used to. Work out with

WEEK 5		WEEK 6	
WEIGHT	**REPS**	**WEIGHT**	**REPS**
20	10	25	8
30	10	35	8
Body	15	Body	15
20	10	25	8

WEEK 8	
WEIGHT	**REPS**
20	8
45	6–8
30	10
25	10

half the weight. Walk or run half the number of miles. After a couple of weeks, you may feel the temptation to start pushing yourself. Don't. Your feet, knees, elbows, and shoulders aren't ready for the pounding, even if your muscles feel great and your stamina seems to be returning. Unfortunately, your joints and connective tissues won't give you any feedback until there's a problem. Instead, increase your miles, speed and weights by 10 percent every week, tops. If you start your program with half of what you were doing before, you can get back to two-thirds within a month. In 2 months, you'll be better than ever.

Your Workout

Do each workout twice a week. The weights specified in the workout charts are just suggestions; they may be too light or heavy. Just make sure you improve each week.

- **Week 1**: do 1 set of each exercise
- **Week 2**: do 2 sets of each exercise
- **Weeks 3–8**: do 3 sets of each exercise

Aerobic Routine

Finish each weight-lifting workout with 30 minutes of your favorite cardiovascular exercise—jogging, cycling or rowing—at a challenging intensity. Three other days a week, do 60 minutes of cardiovascular exercise at a slightly lower intensity; you can do this all at once or break it up—30 minutes before work and 30 minutes after, 20 minutes three times a day, and so forth.

THE 15-MINUTE WORKOUT

A Simple Path to Lean Muscle

This fat-burning workout puts high demands on your energy stores and works your body from several angles. The result: a lean, athletic form. All you need is a 4-pound fitness ball and 15 minutes. Do one exercise after another with 30 to 60 seconds of rest between. Do three circuits 3 days a week, resting at least 1 day between workouts.

REVERSE LUNGE AND BALL TWIST

Targets: Entire Lower Body, Abdominals

1 Stand holding a fitness ball in front of your chest with both hands. Step backward with your left leg and lower your body until your right knee is bent 90 degrees and your left knee nearly touches the floor (in a backward lunge position). Your right lower leg should be perpendicular to the floor. Twist to your right and touch the ball to the floor by leaning over your thigh and straightening your arms.

2 Transfer your body weight to your right leg and push yourself to a standing position as you lift your left knee to your chest.

3 Keeping the knee up, push the ball away from your chest, pull it back quickly, then twist your torso as far as you can to the left.

4 Return to the starting position and repeat 14 times, then switch sides.

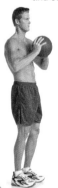
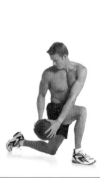
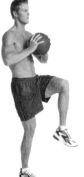
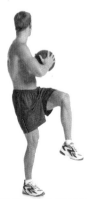

BALL CATCH AND STRADDLE JUMP

Targets: Entire Lower Body

1 Stand holding a fitness ball in front of your chest with both hands, your feet shoulder-width apart. Drop the ball then lower your body into a squat position and catch it after one bounce.

2 As you catch the ball, immediately jump as high as you can and rotate your body 90 degrees to your left.

3 When your feet touch the floor, bounce the ball, squat, and jump to the starting position. Repeat this to the right, and return to the starting position. That's one repetition. Do a total of three repetitions.

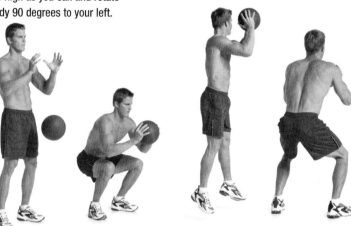

SITUP AND BALL PASS

Targets: Abdominals, Hip Flexors

1 Lie on your back on the floor with your legs bent and feet flat, and hold a fitness ball with your arms straight and horizontal, in line with your body.

2 Raise your head, chest, and right leg at the same time, sweeping your arms forward to lift the ball toward your right foot. Pause when your upper body is at a 45-degree angle from the floor.

3 Move the ball behind your right thigh with one hand and pass it to the other hand and back 10 times.

4 Return to the starting position. Then switch legs and perform the movements again. Repeat one more time with each leg.

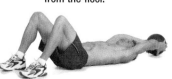
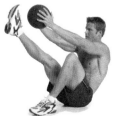
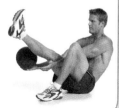

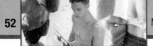

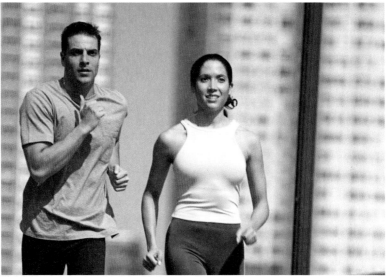

Work out for an hour—burn fat all day. What more could you want?

4-Week Fat-Loss Program

In this 4-week fat-loss program, you'll work your muscles harder than ever before by focusing on total-body movements. So you'll twist when you perform a shoulder press, hoist the barbell as you squat, and stand on one leg when you do bent-over rows. Besides increasing your calorie burn during your exercise session, this strategy also boosts your metabolism for hours afterward. That means you'll burn fat at a higher rate long after your workout is over. You'll also go from one exercise to another with little or no rest between moves. That will trigger a surge in your powerful fat-burning hormones, for an even more effective gut-melting stimulus. Consider this workout your overdue collection notice to that unwanted belly. It's time to make your fat pay.

About Your Workout

This program is divided into two full-body workouts: Workout A and Workout B (see the workout charts on page 54). Alternate between the two, taking a day off after each. So, one week you might do Workout A on Monday and Friday and Workout B on Wednesday, then the following week do Workout B on Monday and Friday and Workout A on Wednesday. Continue in this fashion for the entire 4-week program.

• **Workout A:** The upper-body exercises in Workout A are arranged in supersets—pairs of exercises performed one after the other without rest—instead of straight sets. Complete the moves in the order shown in the charts on the following page. Do all the sets of the Group 1 exercises first, followed by all the sets of the Group 2 exercises, and so on. Do both exercises in each superset without rest.

• **Workout B:** The first two groups of exercises are called "complexes." You do the three exercises in succession without setting down the bar. That's one repetition. (In the second complex, the model is shown using different weights for each phase of the complex, since we originally photographed the moves as stand-alone exercises. But you'll do them using the same weight for each.) Groups 3 and 4 are supersets, just as in Workout A.

Warmup Routine

For each group of exercises, perform a warmup set. Do the number of repetitions suggested with about 60 percent of the weight you'll use for your work sets. Don't exhaust yourself on the warmup sets. They're intended only to prepare your muscles and connective tissues for the harder work to come. You'll reduce your risk of injuries and perform better at the same time.

Abdominal Routine

Perform your favorite abs exercises after each workout—we've included a selection of crunches and twists on pages 78–83. Choose two or three moves and do two or three sets of 10 repetitions of each.

Rest

Rest for 60 seconds after each superset or complex.

Progress

When you can do the maximum number of prescribed repetitions in each set, increase the weight you're using for a particular exercise by 5 to 10 percent.

Workout A

	EXERCISE	REPS
GROUP 1	Squat press (p.57) 25	5–7
GROUP 1	Leg press (p.84)	15–20
GROUP 2	Single-leg alternating dumbbell row (p.58) 75	4–6
GROUP 2	Cable row (p.63) 14	10–15
GROUP 3	Romanian deadlift (p.67) 60	5–7
GROUP 3	Lying leg curl (p.85) 90	10–12
GROUP 4	Swiss ball pushup (p.74) —	6–8
GROUP 4	Barbell bench press (p.71) 30²	10–12
GROUP 5	Dumbbell calf jump (p.92) 25	5–6
GROUP 5	45-degree traveling lunge (p.87) x	10–12
GROUP 6	Twisting shoulder press (p.56) 20	6–10
GROUP 6	Pronated lat pulldown (p.76) 11	10-12

Workout B

	EXERCISE	REPS
COMPLEX 1	Hang clean (p.94)	
COMPLEX 1	Front squat (p.90)	5–8
COMPLEX 1	Barbell push press (p.57)	
COMPLEX 2	Snatch-grip shrug (p.69)	
COMPLEX 2	Romanian deadlift (p.67)	5–8
COMPLEX 2	Bent-over row (p.58)	
GROUP 3	Santana T-pushup (p.75)	6–8
GROUP 3	One-arm lat pulldown (p.77)	10–12
GROUP 4	45-degree traveling lunge (p.87)	8–10
GROUP 4	Dumbbell upright row (p.63)	8–10

PART III
The Exercises

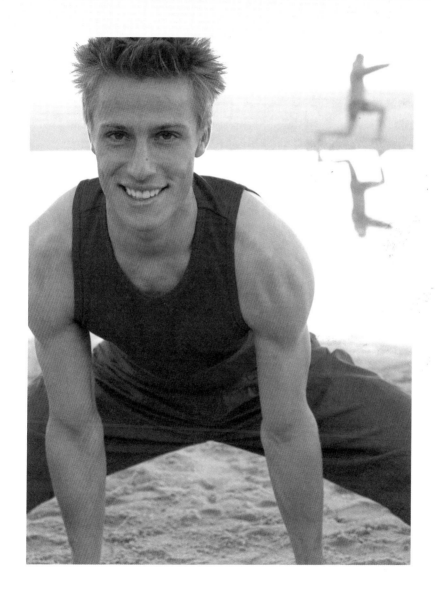

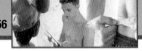
Chest, Back and Arms

Build lean muscle with this collection of upper-body moves.

TWISTING SHOULDER PRESS

■ **Targets:** Deltoids, Triceps, Obliques

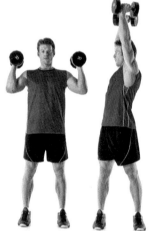

1 Stand holding a pair of dumbbells at the sides of your shoulders, palms turned toward each other, and feet shoulder-width apart.

2 Lift both dumbbells straight over your shoulder as you twist your torso to the right.

3 Lower the weights as you twist back to the starting position, then repeat twisting to your left.

4 If you end the set with an odd number of repetitions, start the next set by twisting to the side opposite the one you finished on in the previous set.

SHOULDER PRESS

■ **Targets:** Deltoids, Triceps, Lower Trapezius

1 Grab a pair of dumbbells and sit on a bench. Hold the dumbbells at the sides of your shoulders, with your arms bent and palms facing each other.

2 Push the weights straight overhead, pause, then slowly lower them.

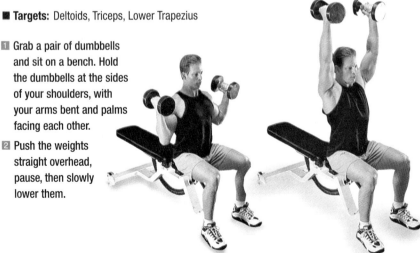

BARBELL PUSH PRESS

■ **Targets:** Deltoids, Triceps, Lower Body

1 Grab a barbell from the rack with an overhand grip that's just beyond shoulder width and position the bar chest high.

2 Bend your knees about 30 to 45 degrees, then quickly and explosively straighten them as you press the bar overhead.

3 Slowly lower the barbell to your shoulders, and immediately perform the next repetition.

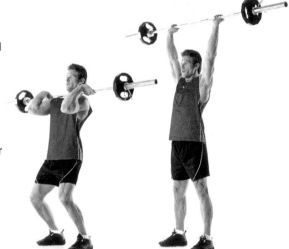

SQUAT PRESS

■ **Targets:** Entire Lower Body, Deltoids, Triceps, all Middle- and Lower-Body Stabilizers

1 Hold a barbell with an overhand grip so that it rests comfortably on your upper back (not on your neck). Set your feet shoulder-width apart, keeping your back straight and eyes focused straight ahead.

2 Slowly lower your body as if you were performing a squat, but keep the bar at the starting level by pushing it up slowly as you squat.

3 When your thighs are parallel to the floor and your arms are fully extended above your shoulders, pause, then return to the starting position.

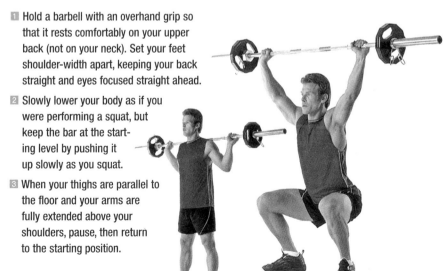

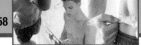

BENT-OVER ROW

■ **Targets:** Trapezius, Lats, Rear Shoulders, Biceps

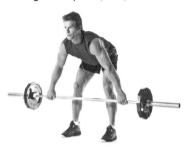
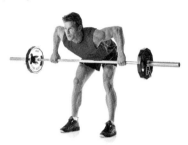

1 Grab a barbell with an overhand grip that's just beyond shoulder-width, and hold it down at arm's length. Stand with your feet shoulder-width apart and knees slightly bent (not pictured).

2 Bend at the hips, lowering your torso about 45 degrees, and let the bar hang straight down from your shoulders.

3 Pull the bar up to your torso, pause, then slowly lower it.

SINGLE-LEG ALTERNATING DUMBBELL ROW

■ **Targets:** Trapezius, Lats, Rear Shoulders, Biceps, all Mid-Body Stabilizers, all Lower Leg Muscles

1 Grab a pair of dumbbells and stand with your left foot in front of your right. Keep your back flat and bend over at the hips so the dumbbells are hanging at arm's length from your shoulders, palms facing in. Raise your right foot off the floor.

2 Raise your left upper arm as high as you can by bending your elbow and squeezing your shoulder blade toward the middle of your back.

3 As you lower it, raise the other—that's one repetition. Alternate until you finish the set.

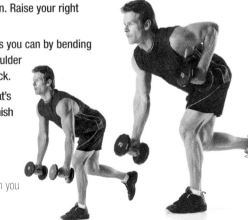

TRAINER'S TIP

Alternate the foot you raise and the arm you start with on each set.

ONE-ARM BENT-OVER ROW

■ **Targets:** Trapezius, Rear Shoulders, Biceps

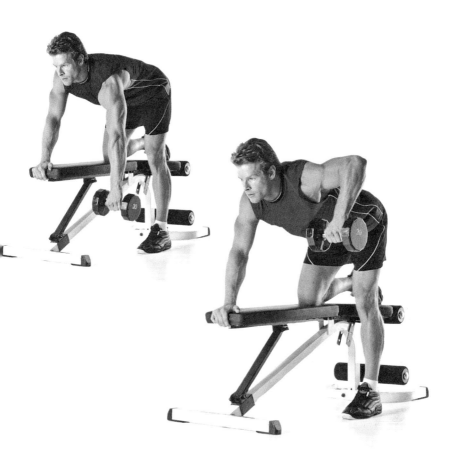

1 Grab a dumbbell in your left hand; place your right hand and right knee on a flat bench. Keep your back flat and your upper body parallel to the floor. Let your left arm hang straight down from your shoulder; turn your palm so that it's facing your left leg.

2 Raise your left upper arm until it's just past parallel to the floor. Your upper arm should be perpendicular to your body at the top of the move. Your lower arm should be pointing toward the floor.

3 Pause, then slowly lower the weight to the starting position.

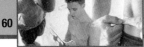

LYING DUMBBELL ROW

■ **Targets:** Trapezius, Rear Shoulders, Biceps

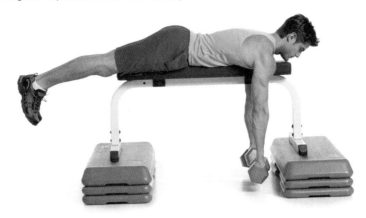

1️⃣ Lie facedown on a high flat bench with your arms hanging straight down holding a dumbbell in each hand.

2️⃣ Row both weights up as far as possible to your sides. Pause and squeeze your shoulder blades together.

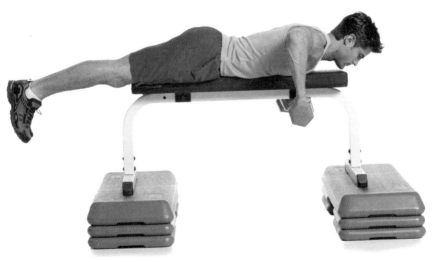

3️⃣ Lower the weights to the starting position and repeat.

TRAINER'S TIP

Keep biceps involvement to a minimum by rowing the weight up to your sides and not up to your chest.

45-DEGREE LYING DUMBBELL ROW

■ **Targets:** Trapezius, Rear Shoulders, Biceps

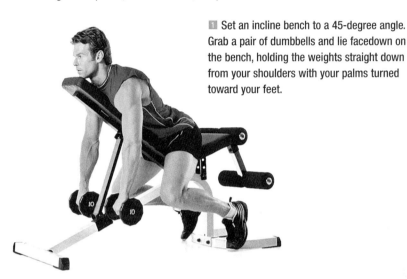

Set an incline bench to a 45-degree angle. Grab a pair of dumbbells and lie facedown on the bench, holding the weights straight down from your shoulders with your palms turned toward your feet.

Lift the weights up and out to your sides so your elbows are bent about 90 degrees and your upper arms are nearly perpendicular to your torso.

Slowly return to the starting position.

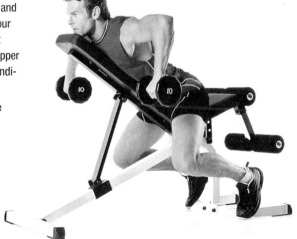

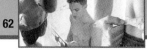

WIDE-GRIP SEATED ROW

■ **Targets:** Lats, Trapezius, Rear Shoulders, Biceps

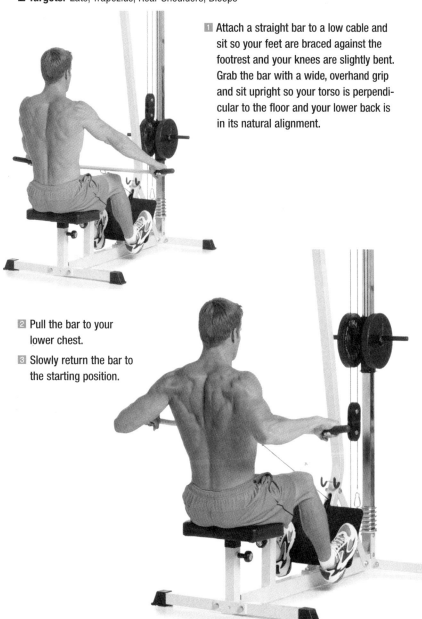

1 Attach a straight bar to a low cable and sit so your feet are braced against the footrest and your knees are slightly bent. Grab the bar with a wide, overhand grip and sit upright so your torso is perpendicular to the floor and your lower back is in its natural alignment.

2 Pull the bar to your lower chest.

3 Slowly return the bar to the starting position.

DUMBBELL UPRIGHT ROW

■ **Targets:** Deltoids, Trapezius

1 Grab a pair of dumbbells with an overhand grip and stand with your feet shoulder-width apart, your knees slightly bent. Let the dumbbells hang at arm's length next to the outside of your thighs, thumbs pointed toward each other.

2 Bending your elbows, lift your upper arms straight out to the sides and pull the dumbbells straight up, until your upper arms are parallel to the floor and the dumbbells are just below chest level. (You'll look like a scarecrow.)

3 Pause, then return to the starting position.

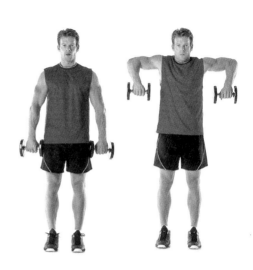

CABLE ROW

■ **Targets:** Lats, Trapezius, Rear Shoulders, Biceps

1 Attach a long, straight bar to the cable and position yourself at the machine. Grab the bar with an overhand grip that's just beyond shoulder-width. Sit up straight; pull your shoulders back.

2 Pull the bar to your abdomen without leaning back more than a few degrees.

3 Pause, then slowly return to the starting position without leaning forward at the waist or hips.

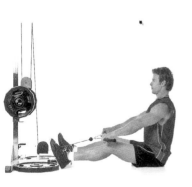

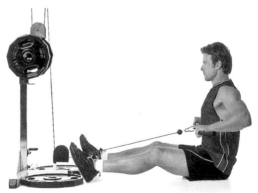

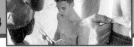

TRICEPS EXTENSION

■ **Targets:** Triceps

1 Grab a pair of dumbbells and sit on the end of a bench with your back straight. Hold the dumbbells at arm's length above your head, your palms facing each other.

2 Without moving your upper arms, lower the dumbbells behind your head until your forearms are just past parallel to the floor.

3 Pause, then straighten your arms to return the dumbbells to the starting position.

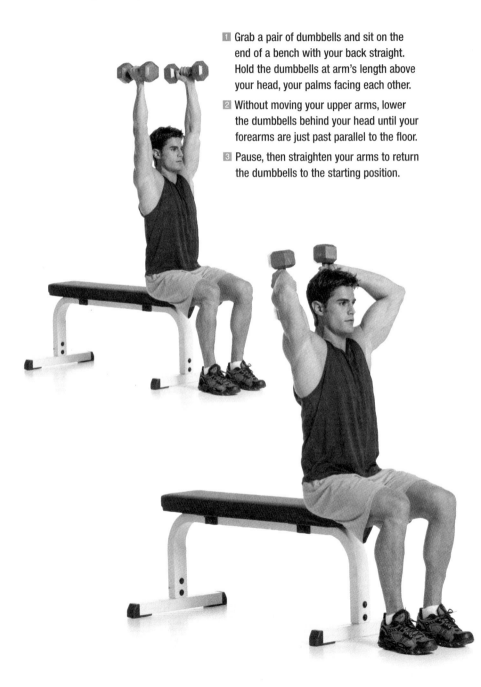

BICEPS CURL

■ **Targets:** Biceps

1. Sit on the end of a bench and hold a dumbbell in each hand with your arms hanging by your sides, palms turned toward your body.
2. Keeping your elbows close to your body, curl the weights forward and up, twisting your palms forward as you lift.
3. Slowly lower the dumbbells, resisting the weight all the way down, until your arms are fully extended.

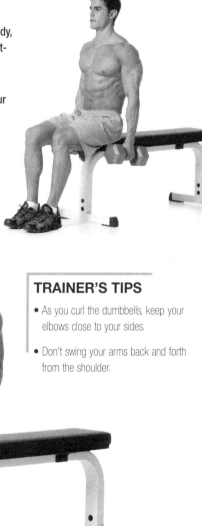

TRAINER'S TIPS

- As you curl the dumbbells, keep your elbows close to your sides.

- Don't swing your arms back and forth from the shoulder.

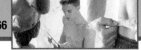

SINGLE-LEG DEADLIFT

■ **Targets:** Hamstrings, Gluteals, Lower Back

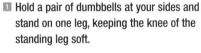

1 Hold a pair of dumbbells at your sides and stand on one leg, keeping the knee of the standing leg soft.

2 Slowly lean forward, keeping your back straight.

3 Slowly return to the starting position, squeezing your gluteals to maintain proper alignment.

TRAINER'S TIP

To avoid straining your lower back, use light dumbbells for this exercise. If you have pre-existing lower-back problems, you may wish to avoid this exercise.

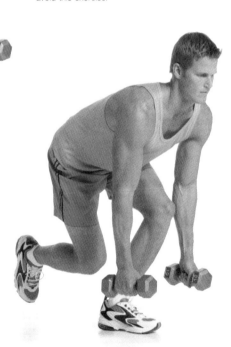

ROMANIAN DEADLIFT

■ **Targets:** Hamstrings, Gluteals, Lower Back

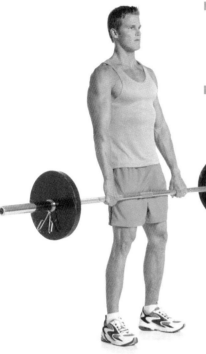

1 Grab a barbell with a wide (but still comfortable) overhand grip. Hold the bar down at arm's length in front of you. Your feet should be hip-width apart and your knees slightly bent.

2 Keep your lower back arched slightly, and slowly bend at the hips as far as you can without losing the arch. (The bar will probably be just below your knees.) Don't change the angle of your knees, and keep the bar as close to your body as possible throughout the movement.

3 Pause, then lift your torso back to the starting position.

TRAINER'S TIP

The Romanian Deadlift is the middle move of a dynamic exercise complex featured in the 4-Week Fat-Loss Program (page 52). Perform the Snatch-Grip Shrug (page 69), Romanian Deadlift, and Bent-Over Row (page 58) in succession without setting the bar down between exercises—that counts as 1 rep.

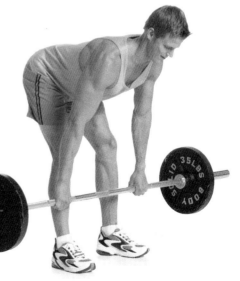

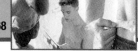

DUMBBELL SHRUG

■ **Targets:** Upper Trapezius

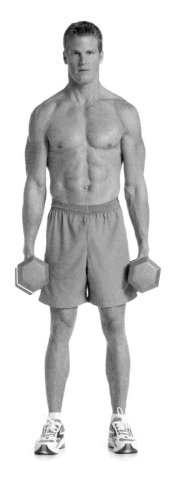

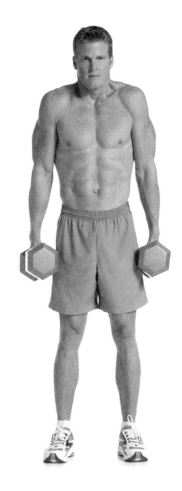

1 Stand with your feet hip-width apart holding dumbbells at your sides, your palms facing your body.

2 Shrug your shoulders toward your ears. Pause, then slowly return to the starting position.

SNATCH-GRIP SHRUG

■ **Targets:** Middle and Upper Trapezius

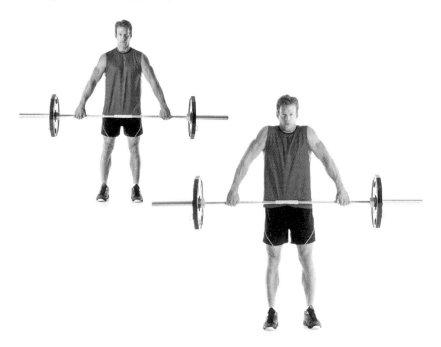

1 Grab a barbell with an overhand grip that's as wide as comfortably possible. Set your feet shoulder-width apart and hold the bar down at arm's length in front of you.

2 Lean forward slightly at the hips so the bar is about an inch in front of your thighs.

3 Shrug your shoulders as high as you can.

4 Pause, then slowly lower the barbell.

TRAINER'S TIP

The Snatch-Grip Shrug is the first of three moves in the dynamic exercise complex featured in the 4-Week Fat-Loss Program (page 52). Perform this exercise, the Romanian Deadlift (page 67), and the Bent-Over Row (page 58) in succession without setting the bar down between exercises—that counts as 1 rep.

Bench Press

The bench press is the granddaddy of all chest exercises, working more muscle fibers in the chest than any other move. Here's the classic bench press plus two variations to help round out your workout. Alternating your hand positions occasionally will help you target different muscle groups—a wider grip emphasizes your chest, while a narrower grip involves more of your triceps and deltoids.

DUMBBELL BENCH PRESS

Targets: Pectorals, Triceps, Front Shoulders

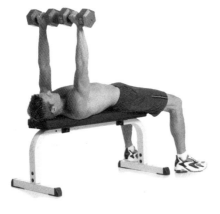

▪ Lie on a flat bench with a dumbbell in each hand (palms forward), your arms extended straight above your chest.

▪ Lower the dumbbells until they're resting along the sides of your chest. Pause, then press the weights back up.

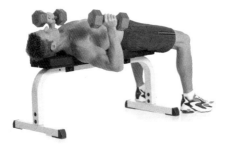

THE DUMBBELL ADVANTAGE

You'll lift less weight with dumbbells, but since they allow your hands to move independently of each other, it will be easier to keep your hands directly in line with your elbows, reducing your risk of injury.

BARBELL BENCH PRESS

Targets: Pectorals, Triceps, Front Shoulders

1 Lie on your back on a flat bench and grab a barbell with an overhand grip, your hands about shoulder-width apart (or as wide as they would be if you were doing a pushup). Hold the bar over your chest with your arms straight.

2 Slowly lower the bar to your chest.

3 Push back up to the starting position.

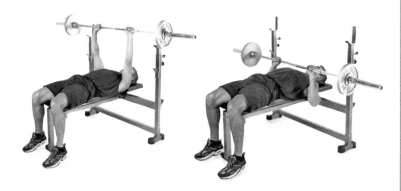

WIDE-GRIP BARBELL BENCH PRESS

Targets: Pectorals, Triceps, Front Shoulders

1 Lie on your back on a flat bench. Grab a barbell with an overhand grip, your hands a bit farther apart than for the barbell bench press, and lift it off the uprights. Hold it over your chin at arm's length.

2 Slowly lower the bar to your chest.

3 Pause, then push the bar back up until your arms are straight and the bar is over your chin again.

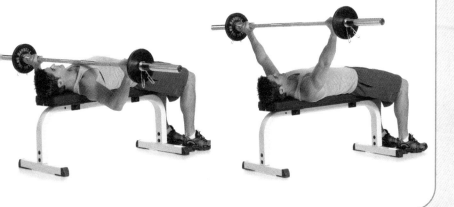

Pushup

The once-forgotten pushup has been reborn as a muscle builder and back saver. Pushups not only build the facade in front of your physique, but also develop the support system behind those muscles, too. So it makes sense that pushups help improve muscular balance, which is important for developing serious strength. And with strength comes muscle size.

PUSHUP

Targets: Pectorals, Triceps, Front Shoulders

1 Get in pushup up position, with your arms about shoulder-width apart. Balance your weight on your toes and palms, with your hands a comfortable distance apart, probably just beyond shoulder-width.

2 Straighten your back by tucking your pelvis.

3 Slowly lower yourself to the floor, pause, and push yourself back up.

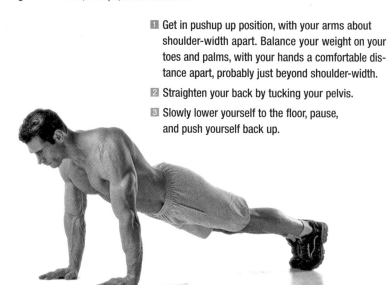

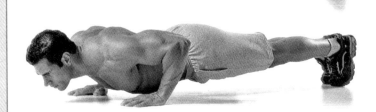

DECLINE PUSHUP

Targets: Pectorals, Triceps, Front Shoulders

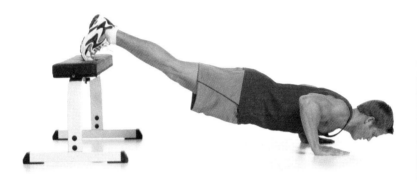

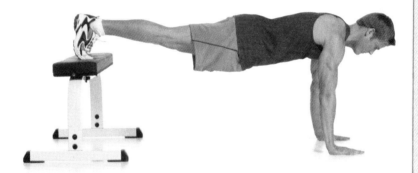

1 Get into pushup position, with hands slightly wider than shoulder-width and feet placed toes-down on a bench or an elevated surface.

2 Keeping your back flat and your head in its natural alignment, slowly push upward from the floor until your arms are almost fully extended.

3 Pause, return to the starting position and repeat.

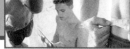

SWISS BALL PUSHUP

■ **Targets:** Pectorals, Triceps, Front Deltoids, all Mid-Body Stabilizers

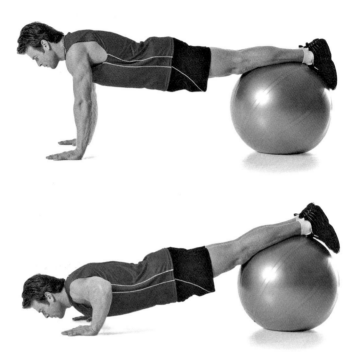

1 Get into pushup position—your hands slightly wider than and in line with your shoulders—but instead of placing your feet on the floor, rest your shins on a Swiss ball. With your arms straight and your back flat, your body should form a straight line from shoulders to ankles.

2 Lower your body until your chest nearly touches the floor.

3 Pause, then push yourself back up to the starting position.

SANTANA T-PUSHUP

■ **Targets:** Pectorals, Triceps, Front and Rear Shoulders, Trapezius, all Mid-Body Stabilizers

1 Get into pushup position with your hands on the handles of dumbbells that have been placed shoulder-width apart.

2 Do a pushup, and as you come up, rotate your body so that you raise your left arm and the dumbbell straight up over your shoulder and your body forms a "T".

3 Lower the dumbbell and yourself, return to the original position, and repeat to the other side.

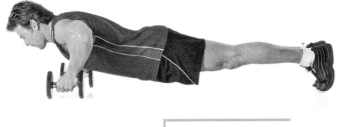

PERFECT YOUR PUSHUP POSTURE

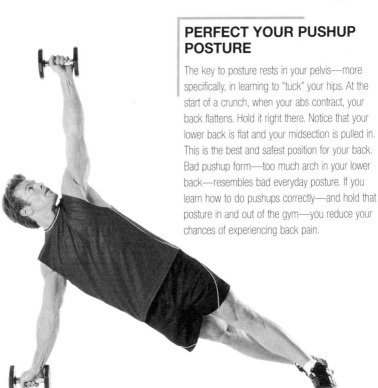

The key to posture rests in your pelvis—more specifically, in learning to "tuck" your hips. At the start of a crunch, when your abs contract, your back flattens. Hold it right there. Notice that your lower back is flat and your midsection is pulled in. This is the best and safest position for your back. Bad pushup form—too much arch in your lower back—resembles bad everyday posture. If you learn how to do pushups correctly—and hold that posture in and out of the gym—you reduce your chances of experiencing back pain.

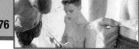

PRONATED LAT PULLDOWN

■ **Targets:** Lats, Trapezius, Rear Shoulders, Biceps

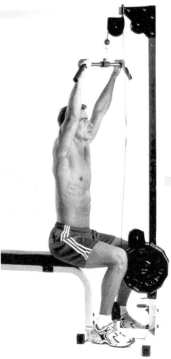

1 Grab the bar overhead with an overhand grip (palms facing away from you), hands just beyond shoulder-width.

2 Sit on the seat and, keeping your head and back straight, slowly pull the bar to the top of your chest. Pause, then let the bar rise back above your head—resisting the weight as you go—until your arms are straight again, but keep your elbows unlocked.

REVERSE YOUR GRIP

Try grabbing the straight bar at the lat pulldown station with an under-hand grip. This variation still builds your upper-back muscles while letting the biceps help curl the bar at the bottom of the move. Also, the position forces the forearms, wrists, and hands to work harder than they have to in most back exercises, helping you develop a stronger grip at the same time.

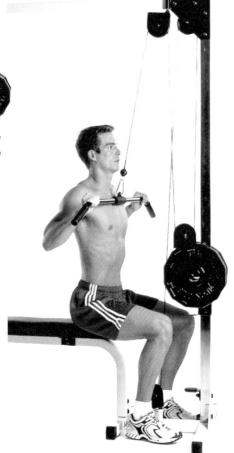

TOWEL PULLDOWN

■ **Targets:** Lats, Trapezius, Biceps, Gripping Muscles

1 Wrap a pair of towels around the bar of a lat-pulldown machine. Position yourself in the machine and grab a towel with each hand, keeping your hands just wider than shoulder-width apart.

2 Pull the bar down to your chest as you lean backward slightly, keeping your back straight.

3 Return to the starting position.

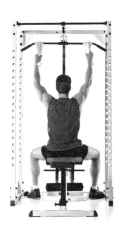
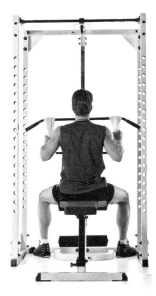

ONE-ARM LAT PULLDOWN

■ **Targets:** Lats, Trapezius, Biceps

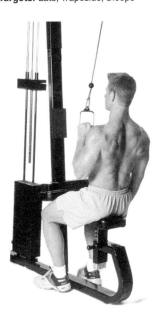

1 Attach a stirrup handle to an overhead cable. Using an overhand grip, grab the handle with one hand (your left if you're right-handed) and position yourself in the machine with your working arm straight and the other down at your side.

2 Pull the handle straight down until it's just outside your chest.

3 Return to the starting position and repeat for the designated number of repetitions. Then, without resting, do the same number with the other arm.

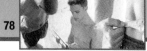

Abdominals

Train your mid-body muscles from every angle.

CRUNCH

■ **Targets:** Rectus Abdominis, Obliques

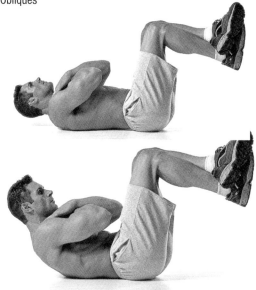

1. Lie on your back with your knees and hips bent about 90 degrees, and cross your arms.

2. Raise your upper body off the floor by crunching your rib cage toward your pelvis. Then lower yourself to the starting position.

TRAINER'S TIP

Where you place your hands can change the degree of difficulty of a crunch. If you can't complete the last repetition of a set, try moving your hands from behind your ears to across your chest. This displaces a portion of your weight and may allow you to do one or two more crunches, to work the muscles a little longer.

SWISS BALL CRUNCH

■ **Targets:** Rectus Abdominis, Obliques

1 Lie on your back on a Swiss ball, with both feet on the floor, just wider than shoulder-width apart. Your head should be slightly lower than your chest. Place your hands behind your ears and point your elbows out.

2 Curl your rib cage toward your pelvis while keeping your head and neck still.

3 Hold, then return to the starting position.

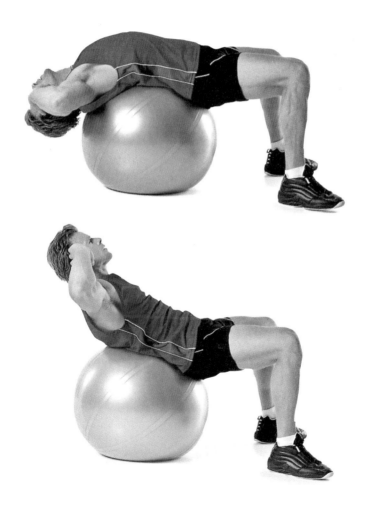

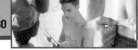

TOWEL CRUNCH

■ **Targets:** Rectus Abdominis, Obliques

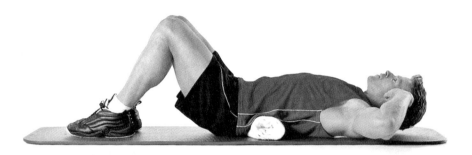

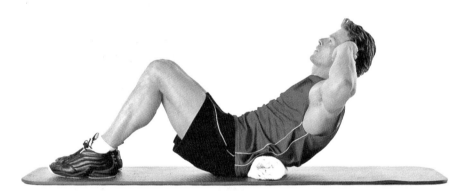

1 Roll up a small towel and lie faceup on the floor with the towel in the arch of your lower back. Place your feet flat on the floor, put your hands behind your ears, and point your elbows out to the sides.

2 Curl your rib cage toward your pelvis, lifting your head and shoulders off the floor.

3 Return to the starting position.

WEIGHTED CRUNCH

■ **Targets:** Rectus Abdominis, Obliques, Hip Flexors

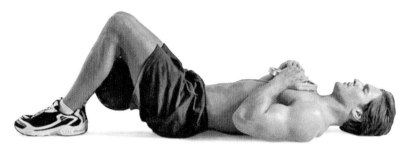

1 Lie flat on your back with your knees bent and your feet flat on the floor. Place a light medicine ball between your knees and squeeze it so it stays in place throughout the exercise. Hold a light weight plate (5 to 8 pounds to start) in your hands.

2 Slowly draw your knees up toward your chest while simultaneously curling your head and shoulders off the ground.

3 Pause, then slowly lower your legs and upper body back to the floor, or just above the floor to keep constant tension on your rectus abdominis.

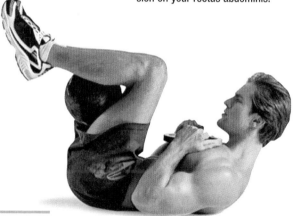

PARTNER UP

Instead of a weight plate, hold a medicine ball at your chest, keeping your elbows out to your sides. Have your workout partner stand in front of you. As you curl up, throw the ball to your partner. Ask him to lightly toss the ball back at your chest so you can catch it, pull it back to your body, and then curl back down.

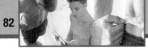

TWISTING LEGS-UP CRUNCH

■ **Targets:** Rectus Abdominis, Obliques

1 Lie on your back and raise your legs so that the soles of your feet point toward the ceiling.

2 Place your hands lightly behind your ears, elbows pointing out. Keeping your legs upright, slowly curl up and to the left.

3 Lower yourself and repeat to the right. Alternate from left to right throughout the set.

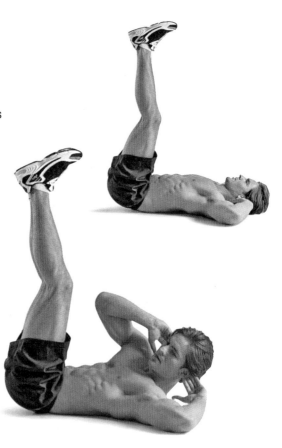

GET MORE

Start the move with your legs straight and suspended at a 45-degree angle to the floor. As you curl your upper body off the floor, simultaneously raise your legs until your feet point toward the ceiling. As you bring your head and shoulders back down to the floor, lower your legs back to a 45-degree angle.

PULSE TWIST

■ **Targets:** Rectus Abdominis, Obliques

[1] Lie on your back and tuck your hands under your pelvis, along the sides of your tailbone.

[2] Keeping your legs straight and feet together, raise them so the soles of your feet point toward the ceiling and your buttocks lift a few inches off the floor. At the top of the move, twist your hips to the right so that your feet point to the left.

[3] Lower your legs back to the starting position and repeat the move, this time twisting your hips to the left.

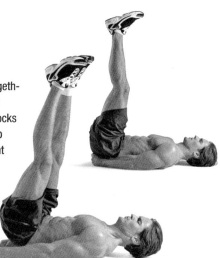

PUSHUP BRIDGE

■ **Targets:** All Mid-Body Stabilizers

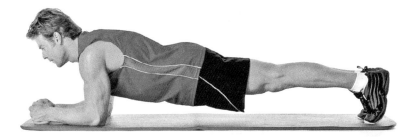

[1] Start to get into a pushup position, but bend your elbows and rest your weight on your forearms instead of your hands. Your body should form a straight line from your shoulders to your ankles.

[2] Pull in your abdominals; imagine you're trying to move your belly button back to your spine. Hold for 20 to 30 seconds, breathing steadily.

[3] Release, then repeat for another 20 to 30 seconds. That equals two complete sets. As you build endurance, you can do one 60-second set instead of two shorter ones.

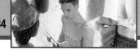
Legs

Build a powerful, chiseled lower body with these dynamic moves

LEG PRESS

■ **Targets:** Quadriceps

1 Position yourself in a leg-press machine with your feet slightly wider than shoulder-width apart and toward the top of the platform. (Use the position that's most comfortable for your knees.) Straighten your legs without locking your knees.

2 Release the supports, then lower the platform until your legs are just past a 90-degree angle. Keep your lower back against the pad throughout the movement.

3 Push the platform back to the starting position.

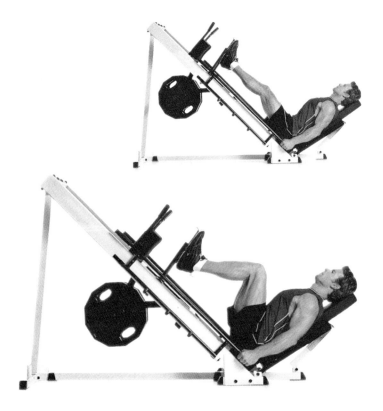

LYING LEG CURL

■ **Targets:** Hamstrings

1 Lie facedown on a leg-curl machine with the pads against your lower legs, above your heels and below your calf muscles.

2 Without raising your body off the pads, bend your knees and pull the weight toward you as far as you can.

3 Pause, then slowly return to the starting position.

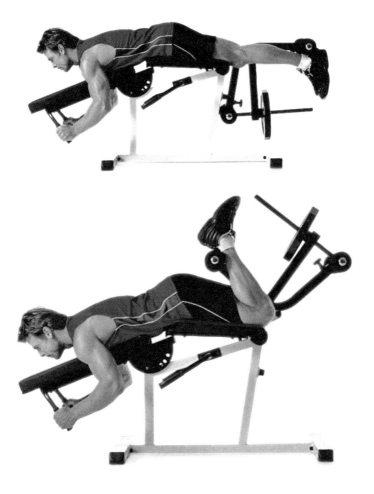

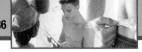
DUMBBELL LUNGE

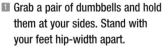

■ **Targets:** Entire Lower Body

1 Grab a pair of dumbbells and hold them at your sides. Stand with your feet hip-width apart.

2 Step forward with your nondominant leg (your left if you're right-handed) and lower your body until your front knee is bent 90 degrees and your other knee nearly touches the floor.

3 Push yourself back up quickly and repeat with your dominant leg forward.

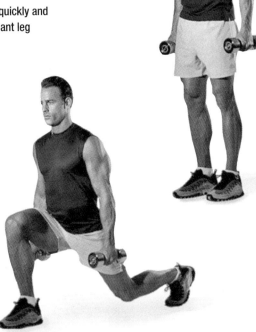

TRAINER'S TIPS

• Make sure your front knee never extends beyond your toes throughout the exercise.

• Bending your rear knee as your forward foot hits the ground will strengthen your quadriceps. It will also prevent your front knee from extending too far.

45-DEGREE TRAVELING LUNGE

■ **Targets:** Entire Lower Body

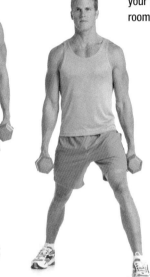

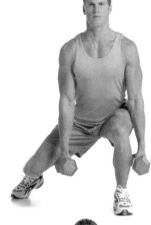

1 Grab a pair of dumbbells and hold them at your sides. Stand with your feet hip-width apart at one end of your house or the gym; you need room to walk forward 16 to 20 steps.

2 Step forward with your left foot at a 45-degree angle; lower your body so your right thigh is perpendicular to the floor and your left knee is bent 90 degrees. Your right knee should also bend and almost touch the floor.

3 Stand and bring your right foot up next to your left, then repeat with the right leg lunging forward at a 45-degree angle. That's one repetition.

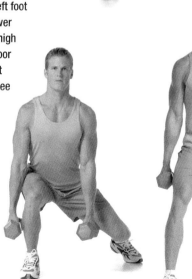

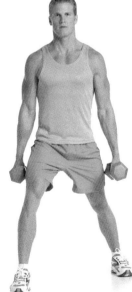

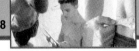

DUMBBELL SQUAT

■ **Targets:** Entire Lower Body

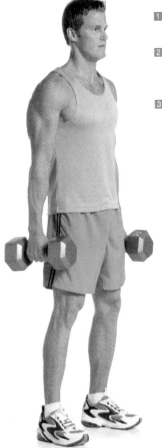

1 Stand with feet shoulder-width apart, holding a dumb-bell in each hand.

2 Bend your knees and lower your body until your thighs are parallel to the floor, making sure your knees do not go over your toes.

3 Pause, then push back to the starting position.

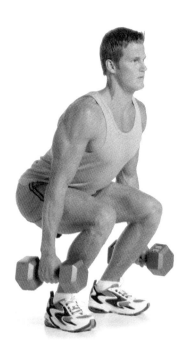

TRAINER'S TIPS

• Keep your head up, eyes focused straight ahead.

• Stand with your shoulders pulled back, your chest out, and your back naturally arched.

• Keep your knees slightly bent and your feet shoulder-width apart.

• On your way down, your knees should track in the same direction your toes are pointing.

BARBELL SQUAT

■ **Targets:** Entire Lower Body

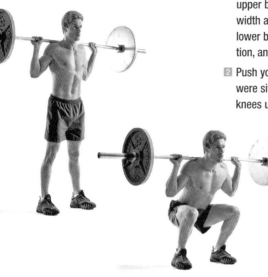

1. Stand holding a barbell across your upper back. Set your feet shoulder-width apart, toes pointed forward, lower back in its naturally arched position, and eyes focused straight ahead.

2. Push your hips backward, as if you were sitting in a chair, and bend your knees until your thighs are slightly below parallel to the floor.

3. Stand back up to the starting position.

DUMBBELL SPLIT SQUAT

■ **Targets:** Entire Lower Body

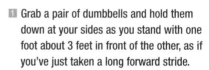

1. Grab a pair of dumbbells and hold them down at your sides as you stand with one foot about 3 feet in front of the other, as if you've just taken a long forward stride.

2. Lower your body until the top of your forward thigh is parallel to the floor and your rear knee almost touches the floor.

3. Return to the starting position. Finish the set, then repeat with your other leg forward.

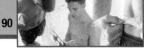

FRONT SQUAT

■ **Targets:** Entire Lower Body

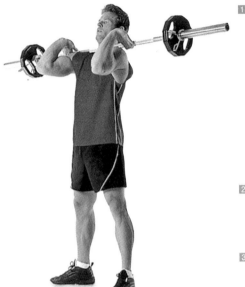

1 Grab a barbell with an overhand grip, hands just beyond shoulder-width, and hold it in front of you, just above the shoulders. Raise your upper arms so they're parallel to the floor while letting the bar roll back onto your fingers. Your feet should be shoulder-width apart, knees slightly bent. Keep your back straight.

2 Without changing the position of your arms, lower your body until your thighs are parallel to the floor.

3 Pause, then push back to the starting position.

TRAINER'S TIP

The Front Squat is the middle move of a dynamic exercise complex featured in the 4-Week Fat-Loss Program (page 52). Perform the Hang Clean (page 94), Front Squat, and Barbell Push Press (page 57) in succession without setting the bar down between exercises—that counts as 1 rep.

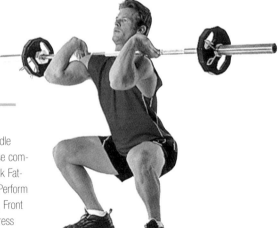

DUMBBELL STEPUP

■ **Targets:** Entire Lower Body

1 Grab a pair of dumbbells and stand in front of a bench or step that's 12 to 18 inches high.

2 Step up onto the bench with your right foot and push off with your right heel to lift the rest of your body onto the step. Step down with your left foot first, then your right.

3 Finish the set with your right leg, then repeat the set with your left leg, stepping up with your left and back with your right.

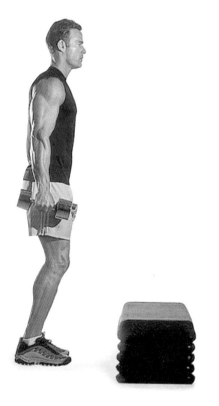
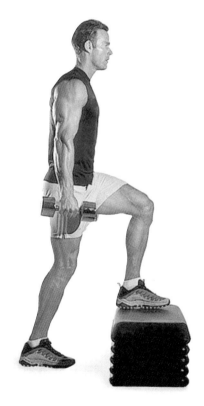

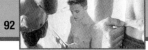

DUMBBELL CALF JUMP

■ **Targets:** Calves

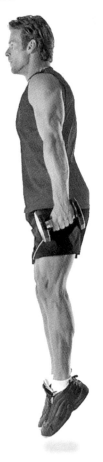

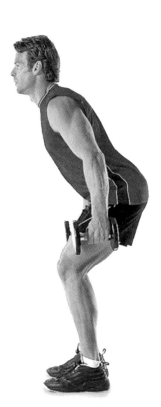

1 Standing with your feet hip-width apart, grab a pair of dumbbells and hold them down at your sides at arm's length.

2 Dip your knees so they're bent about 45 degrees, and jump as high as you can. Point your toes straight down to the floor when you jump.

3 Allow your knees to bend 45 degrees when you land, then immediately jump and point your toes again.

FARMER'S WALK ON TOES

■ **Targets:** Calves, Gripping Muscles in Hands and Forearms

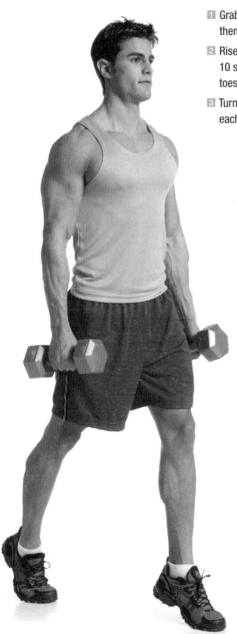

1 Grab a pair of dumbbells and hold them at your sides.

2 Rise on your toes and walk forward 10 steps with each leg. Stay on your toes the entire time.

3 Turn and walk back 10 steps with each leg.

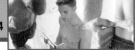

GOOD MORNING

■ **Targets:** Hamstrings, Gluteals, Lower Back

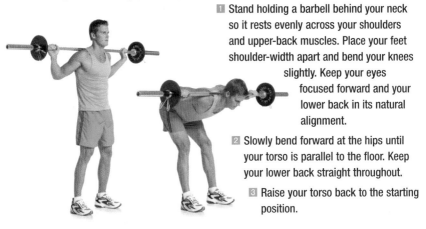

1 Stand holding a barbell behind your neck so it rests evenly across your shoulders and upper-back muscles. Place your feet shoulder-width apart and bend your knees slightly. Keep your eyes focused forward and your lower back in its natural alignment.

2 Slowly bend forward at the hips until your torso is parallel to the floor. Keep your lower back straight throughout.

3 Raise your torso back to the starting position.

HANG CLEAN

■ **Targets:** Hamstrings, Gluteals, Lower Back, Trapezius

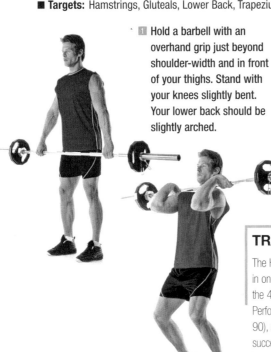

1 Hold a barbell with an overhand grip just beyond shoulder-width and in front of your thighs. Stand with your knees slightly bent. Your lower back should be slightly arched.

2 Shrug your shoulders; pull the bar up as hard as you can while rising up on your toes. When the bar reaches chest level, bend your knees, rotate your upper arms under the bar, and bend your wrists so they go around the bar as you "catch" it on the front of your shoulders.

TRAINER'S TIP

The Hang Clean is the first of three moves in one of the dynamic exercise complex of the 4-Week Fat-Loss Program (page 52). Perform the Hang Clean, Front Squat (page 90), and Barbell Push Press (page 57) in succession without setting the bar down between exercises for 1 rep.

INDEX